MCQs in psychiatry for medical students

John Lally & John Tully

RCPsych Publications

© The Royal College of Psychiatrists 2016

RCPsych Publications is an imprint of the Royal College of Psychiatrists,
21 Prescot Street, London E1 8BB
http://www.rcpsych.ac.uk

British Library Cataloguing-in-Publication Data.
A catalogue record for this book is available from the British Library.
ISBN 978-1-909726-48-2

Distributed in North America by Publishers Storage and Shipping Company.

The views presented in this book do not necessarily reflect those of the Royal College of
Psychiatrists, and the publishers are not responsible for any error of omission or fact.

The Royal College of Psychiatrists is a charity registered in England and Wales (228636)
and in Scotland (SC038369).

Printed by Bell & Bain Ltd, Glasgow, UK

Contents

Foreword

Given their high reliability, ease of implementation, and the comprehensive range of material they can assess, multiple choice questions (MCQs) and extended matching item (EMI) questions increasingly comprise the main knowledge assessments in medical schools. It is crucial, therefore, that students wishing to prepare for such examinations have plenty of exposure to the style and content of these assessments.

The authors of this helpful book are both clinical academics who commenced their psychiatry training in Galway and subsequently moved to academic posts in London. Their experience in undergraduate teaching and curricular development emerges in the comprehensive span and careful construction of the questions in this book. In contrast to the brief stems and checklist-style memorization that characterised older MCQ exam preparation materials, the questions in this book are clinically orientated and have narrative stems in keeping with modern developments in medical education for the clinical years of medical school. Students will need to synthesise and integrate clinical information to arrive at the best answers, and this will facilitate deeper learning. The depth of learning is enhanced by the comprehensive explanations and context provided by the authors in the answers, along with recommendations for further reading on each topic.

This book is a valuable resource for medical students in developing their knowledge of psychiatry and preparing for assessments. As well as testing the student's current knowledge, it will help to identify areas of weakness and to plan future learning. It will also be of interest to postgraduate trainees in psychiatry and more senior clinicians, who would find it educational to dip into this core material for their own interest and revision. The authors are to be commended for the high quality of this work, a substantial support to psychiatry learning for the modern medical student.

Colm McDonald, Professor of Psychiatry
National University of Ireland, Galway, Ireland

Introduction

A solid understanding of psychiatry is a fundamental part of becoming a doctor. As well as providing a platform for future psychiatrists, knowledge of psychiatric disorders is critical for other doctors. Up to 25% of all GP consultations have a mental health component and doctors in other specialties will inevitably encounter psychiatric problems in their day-to-day practice.

Undergraduate psychiatry in the UK is taught by a combination of tutorials, lectures, access to clinical meetings and one-to-one interviews with patients. This system aims to provide a range of experience that will develop a student's understanding of the biological, psychological and social components of psychiatric disorders. Knowledge and skills are assessed by a number of methods. One of these is the objective structured clinical examination (OSCE), which tests the student's communication skills and ability to apply basic knowledge. These examinations are well covered by textbooks and training courses.

However, the other core aspect of medical-student examinations in psychiatry – the multiple choice question – is underserved by currently available textbooks. Many of those available feature outdated 'true–false' questions and few include more modern extended matching item (EMI) questions. Examples of 'best of five' multiple-choice questions (MCQs), which form the backbone of most undergraduate exams, are often not in keeping with the latest research and clinical concepts in psychiatry, and lack appropriate references.

In this book, we seek to address this issue by providing an up-to-date and comprehensively referenced source of questions for medical students in psychiatry. Students will find the format of the questions very much in keeping with the current style of written examinations in their universities.

We anticipate that students will find this an easy-to-use and reliable book that will help them optimise their performance in exams. Further, we hope it will serve as a source of stimulation towards further training and a career in the fascinating specialty of psychiatry. Finally, we believe it will also be of interest to postgraduate trainees in psychiatry in their preparation for membership exams, and to more senior clinicians for the purposes of revision.

How to use this book

This book contains 'best of five' MCQs and EMI questions. The questions are divided into chapters according to subject. These questions are pitched at the level of a testing university examination, with some perhaps above the level required to pass. Self-testing with such a level of difficulty will help students optimise their performance in exams.

The questions are then repeated with the correct answer highlighted, and explanations and references provided. The explanations and references will suffice for students wishing to clarify core concepts and consolidate their learning. The core texts used as references for many of the answers are among the most widely used and highly regarded sources in psychiatry today.

For those interested in exploring the topic in more depth, the suggestions for further reading are up-to-date guide towards more detailed material. Many of these sources are academic papers and clinical guidelines that undergraduate students would not be expected to know in order to pass exams. However, they will help the student develop a deeper understanding of contemporary psychiatry, psychology and neuroscience.

Common abbreviations and terms

ADHD   Attention-deficit hyperactivity disorder
APA   American Psychiatric Association
BMI   Body mass index
EMI   Extended matching item
GP   General practitioner
HDL   High-density lipoprotein
LSD   Lysergic acid diethylamide
MCQ   Multiple-choice question
MMSE   Mini-Mental State Examination
NICE   National Institute for Health and Care Excellence
OCD   Obsessive–compulsive disorder
PTSD   Post-traumatic stress disorder
SNRI   Serotonin–norepinephrine reuptake inhibitor
SSRI   Selective serotonin-reuptake inhibitor
WHO   World Health Organization

Acknowledgements

John Lally would like to thank his parents, Frank & Monica, for inspiring his passion for learning and knowledge and for their continuing support.

John Tully would like to thank all his family for their support and encouragement, and dedicate this book to his mother Ann and his late father Tim.

Both authors would like to thank all those who have provided professional support, guidance and encouragement.

CHAPTER 1

Psychopathology

MCQs

1   A 24-year-old man describes a belief that MI5 is monitoring his thoughts by means of a microchip, which has been inserted in his head and is being used to remove his thoughts and transfer them to their computer system. He remains adamant about this belief in repeated interviews. What first-rank symptom of schizophrenia is he describing?

(a)   Thought insertion
(b)   Delusion of control
(c)   Third-person auditory hallucination
(d)   Thought withdrawal
(e)   Thought broadcasting

2   You assess a 26-year-old woman with a diagnosis of bipolar disorder in the emergency department. She is speaking very quickly and is difficult to interrupt. She scarcely finishes a sentence before starting another. She speaks about a range of topics, but her words make sense and the topics are clearly linked to one another. What sign is she exhibiting?

(a)   Pressure of speech
(b)   Dysphasia
(c)   Tangentiality
(d)   Alogia
(e)   Circumstantiality

3   A 45-year-old man with a diagnosis of paranoid schizophrenia is asked about his personal background. He replies to each question by providing a wealth of information, some of which is only loosely related to the question asked. It is difficult to persuade him to get to the point and to elicit the complete history, although eventually he does meaningfully answer each question. Which term most accurately describes this phenomenon?

(a)   Tangentiality
(b)   Circumstantiality
(c)   Loosening of association
(d)   Thought block
(e)   Derailment

4   You are assessing a 19-year-old man in an in-patient unit. His thinking seems slow, although he is answering questions. On several occasions, however, he stops mid-sentence and seems unable to recall what he was saying. He tells you that he thinks that another patient is stopping his thoughts. Which term most accurately describes this?

(a)   Tangentiality
(b)   Thought withdrawal
(c)   Loosening of association
(d)   Thought block
(e)   Derailment

5   A 54-year-old man with paranoid schizophrenia becomes highly agitated on the ward. You are asked to assess him, but he refuses to come to an interview room. He speaks loudly at you and you can make out his words. However, you cannot elicit any connection between his thoughts. His speech seems jumbled and contains words such as 'wigwag' and 'homo tapean'. Which term most accurately describes his behaviour?

(a)   Tangentiality with speech invention
(b)   Derailment with neologisms
(c)   Thought broadcasting
(d)   Thought insertion with dysphasia
(e)   Thought withdrawal with pressured speech

6   A 34-year-old man believes that his neighbours are trying to force him to leave his property. He believes they are sending threatening messages in Morse code through the radiators in his apartment. He also believes they are taunting him by having a small English flag on their car during the World Cup, as he is originally from Poland. He is adamant that he is correct despite you offering alternative and more likely explanations. How would you classify the nature of his beliefs?

(a)   Persecutory delusions
(b)   Grandiose delusions
(c)   Delusions of control
(d)   Over-valued ideas
(e)   Thought insertion

7   A 54-year-old woman with a history of bipolar disorder complains that nursing staff on the ward are interfering with her 'special mission' to rid the city of sin. She says she should be allowed to leave the ward and continue her good work. She says she knows she has been chosen by God to do this work as when she prays, she feels 'full of energy and love'. Her husband tells you that although she attends church regularly, these beliefs are new and out of character for her. How would you describe her beliefs?

(a)   Nihilistic delusions
(b)   Delusions of prayer
(c)   Delusions of power
(d)   Over-valued ideas
(e)   Religious delusions

8   A 23-year-old man believes that his bowels are being twisted by an alien force that originated on Mars but now lives in Malta. What feature of this delusion makes it more likely that his diagnosis is schizophrenia?

(a)   It involves aliens
(b)   It involves Malta
(c)   It is bizarre
(d)   It is a primary delusion
(e)   It involves his bowels

9   A 43-year-old father of three believes his wife is having an affair. He has been examining her laundry and trying to access her email account. There is no basis in reality to his belief and he has no proof to support it. However, he is adamant that he is correct. His wife has tried to reassure him but she feels this is just making it worse. What is this man's diagnosis?

(a)   Delusion of love
(b)   Morbid jealousy
(c)   Sexual envy disorder
(d)   Delusion of control
(e)   Erotomania

10 A 65-year-old woman tells you at the out-patient clinic that her husband has been replaced by a double. This person looks the same as her husband and shares the same mannerisms as him, but in her view is certainly not her husband. How would you describe her beliefs?

(a)   Folie à deux
(b)   Delusional infidelity
(c)   Delusional interpretation
(d)   Capgras syndrome
(e)   Delusional memory

11 A 57-year-old man believes the electricity company is persecuting him by sending error messages on a website and by making the lights flicker on and off at night. As there is no evidence, his wife initially does not believe him, but over time comes to share his belief. What is this phenomenon called?

(a) Folie à deux
(b) Delusions of control
(c) Delusional interpretation
(d) Delusions of infestation
(e) Fregoli syndrome

12 A 33-year-old woman with paranoid schizophrenia describes hearing voices when there is no one around. They are both male and female and they tell her to harm others. She finds them very distressing and it is difficult for her to resist acting on them. How would you describe this symptom?

(a) Sensory distortion
(b) Third-person auditory hallucination
(c) Second-person command auditory hallucination
(d) Pseudohallucination
(e) Autoscopic hallucination

13 A 23-year-old man describes hearing voices inside his head, talking about him. They say things like 'I think he should harm himself' and also argue between themselves. He cannot dismiss the voices at will. The voices seem real. How would you describe this symptom?

(a) Pseudohallucination
(b) Third-person auditory hallucination
(c) Running commentary
(d) Sensory distortion
(e) Illusion

14 A 19-year-old college student who has been drinking and taking drugs regularly for several weeks is admitted to hospital feeling unwell. Within a day, he develops the sensation of insects crawling inside his skin. There is no evidence that there are insects there. What is the correct term for his symptom?

(a) Olfactory hallucination
(b) Visual hallucination
(c) Auditory hallucination
(d) Gustatory hallucination
(e) Formication

15 A 68-year-old man has cognitive impairment and Parkinsonism, but no history of schizophrenia. He complains of seeing spiders in his room during the day over the course of several weeks. He describes them in great detail and seems frightened of them. There is no evidence that there are spiders in his room. What do you think is the most likely cause for this symptom?

(a) Old age
(b) Dementia with Lewy bodies
(c) Schizophrenia
(d) Alzheimer's disease
(e) Depression

16 A 72-year-old woman is asked to immediately repeat back three words that are said to her in the MMSE. What component of memory does this test?

(a) Short-term memory
(b) Recall
(c) Medium-term memory
(d) Long-term memory
(e) Registration

17 A consultant asks one of her patients, who has a diagnosis of schizophrenia, whether or not the patient believes he has an illness. She asks him if he needs medication and if he needs to stay in hospital. What part of the mental state examination is this?

(a) Memory tests
(b) Investigation of knowledge
(c) Test of attention
(d) Investigating insight
(e) Developing rapport

EMI questions

Thought disorder

Options:

    (a) Flight of ideas
    (b) Thought block
    (c) Derailment
    (d) Tangentiality
    (e) Thought insertion
    (f) Circumstantiality
    (g) Thought withdrawal
    (h) Thought broadcasting

From the list above, select the correct symptom for each of the scenarios below.

1 A 35-year-old man with schizophrenia is speaking very quickly and jumps from subject to subject. There seems to be no connection between his thoughts and what he says does not make any sense to you.

2 A 28-year-old woman with bipolar disorder speaks very quickly, going from subject to subject. She goes off track on each subject before starting again and does not get back to her original topic.

3 A 56-year-old woman with delirium develops depressive psychosis. She believes the nursing staff are 'stealing' thoughts from her head using equipment in her hospital room.

Types of delusion

Options:

    (a) Delusions of grandeur
    (b) Delusions of infestation
    (c) Persecutory delusions
    (d) Capgras syndrome
    (e) Delusions of infidelity
    (f) Folie à deux
    (g) Nihilistic delusions
    (h) Erotomania

From the list above, select the correct term for each of the delusions below.

1 A 22-year-old man believes the police are watching him on camera. He thinks they are doing this as they have an agenda to harm him and send him to prison. There is no evidence that this is the case.

2   A 48-year-old man has a long-standing belief that he is infected with lice. He cannot see or feel the lice but he says he 'just know[s] they are there'. There is no evidence this is the case. He persists in this belief despite being otherwise well.

3   A 20-year-old woman believes that a Member of Parliament (whom she has never met) is in love with her. She believes she has to be with him or her life will be over and goes to extreme lengths to make this happen.

Memory problems

Options:

- (a)   Working memory
- (b)   Semantic memory
- (c)   Implicit memory
- (d)   Registration deficit
- (e)   Confabulation
- (f)   Declarative memory
- (g)   Recall deficit
- (h)   Anterograde memory loss
- (i)   Autobiographical memory

From the list above, select the area of deficit and/or type of deficit for each of the cases below. There is more than one correct answer for some of the scenarios.

1   A 72-year-old man only remembers one of the three items read to him on the MMSE, although he was able to repeat them back to you initially. (Select one option.)

2   A 54-year-old man who has been involved in a road traffic accident has a memory deficit for what happened for 24 h after the event. (Select one option.)

3   An 85-year-old woman with advanced Alzheimer's disease cannot recall many details from the last few years of her life or the name of the current Prime Minister. (Select two options.)

4   A 35-year-old athlete who had a head injury struggles on tests of cognitive performance. When asked about recent events he cannot recall, he 'fills in the gaps', giving false information. (Select one option.)

MCQ answers

1 A 24-year-old man describes a belief that MI5 is monitoring his thoughts by means of a microchip that has been inserted in his head, which is used to remove his thoughts and transfer them to their computer system. He remains adamant about this belief in repeated interviews. What first-rank symptom of schizophrenia is he describing?

    (a)   Thought insertion
    (b)   Delusion of control
    (c)   Third-person auditory hallucination
    (d)   **Thought withdrawal**
    (e)   Thought broadcasting

Kurt Schneider was a German psychiatrist who contributed significantly to the diagnostics of mental disorders. He proposed first-rank symptoms that were more characteristic of schizophrenia than of other psychoses. These consist of three types of auditory hallucinations (hearing one's thoughts out loud, 'running commentary' and two or more voices heard arguing/discussing), delusions of control of impulse/affect/volition/the body, 'thought interference' (external interference with one's thoughts) and delusional perception (delusional interpretation of a normal perception). Thought withdrawal is a form of thought interference (the others being thought insertion and thought broadcasting), which is a belief that one's thoughts are being 'taken or 'stolen' from one's mind.

The validity of first-rank symptoms as a diagnostic or prognostic indicator in schizophrenia has been a subject of debate for decades. It has been long established that first-rank symptoms can occur in other conditions and schizophrenia can occur in the absence of first-rank symptoms. Research continues to sound a note of caution but also points to ongoing relevance. See Oyebode (2008) and, for further reading, Rosen *et al* (2011).

2 You assess a 26-year-old woman with a diagnosis of bipolar disorder in the emergency department. She is speaking very quickly and is difficult to interrupt. She scarcely finishes a sentence before starting another. She speaks about a range of topics, but her words make sense and the topics are clearly linked to one another. What sign is she exhibiting?

    (a)   **Pressure of speech**
    (b)   Dysphasia
    (c)   Tangentiality
    (d)   Alogia
    (e)   Circumstantiality

This woman is exhibiting pressure of speech, a common feature of manic or hypomanic episodes. It is often accompanied by flight of ideas, which is an acceleration in the flow of thinking with little focus on the 'goal' of thinking, although with maintenance of logical connections between thoughts. See Oyebode (2008).

3 A 45-year-old man with a diagnosis of paranoid schizophrenia is asked about his personal background. He replies to each question by providing a wealth of information, some of which is only loosely related to the question asked. It is difficult to persuade him to get to the point and elicit the complete history, although eventually he does meaningfully answer each question. Which term most accurately describes this phenomenon?

    (a)   Tangentiality
    (b)   **Circumstantiality**
    (c)   Loosening of association
    (d)   Thought block
    (e)   Derailment

Circumstantiality is an abnormality in the form of thought often seen in patients with a psychotic illness. It may also be found in those with epilepsy, other organic states, learning difficulties and obsessional personalities and in those with no evidence of mental illness. Excessive and unnecessary information is provided before relevant information is given, obscuring the real answers to questions. However it differs from tangentiality (replying to a question in an oblique and even irrelevant manner), in that the patient does eventually get to the point. See Oyebode (2008) and, for further reading, Swinkels *et al* (2005).

4 You are assessing a 19-year-old man in an in-patient unit. His thinking seems slow, although he is answering questions. On several occasions, however, he stops mid-sentence and seems unable to recall what he was saying. He tells you that he thinks that another patient is stopping his thoughts. Which term most accurately describes this?

    (a)   Tangentiality
    (b)   Thought withdrawal
    (c)   Loosening of association
    (d)   **Thought block**
    (e)   Derailment

This is thought block, which occurs in schizophrenia. The person has the experience of their thoughts 'snapping off', which is followed by an unexpected silence. The person might then begin speaking again about an entirely different topic, without any embarrassment or acknowledgement that a pause had occurred. For others who retain some insight, this can be a very distressing and terrifying experience.

The person might have a belief that someone or something is responsible for the thought blocking: in this case, the man believes that another patient is doing it. This is a 'secondary delusion' (i.e. a delusional belief arising from a 'primary' symptom – in this case, thought block). See Oyebode (2008).

5   A 54-year-old man with paranoid schizophrenia becomes highly agitated on the ward. You are asked to assess him, but he refuses to come to an interview room. He speaks loudly at you and you can make out his words. However, you cannot elicit any connection between his thoughts. His speech seems jumbled and contains words such as 'wigwag' and 'homo tapean'. Which term most accurately describes his behaviour?

   (a)   Tangentiality with speech invention
   (b)   **Derailment with neologisms**
   (c)   Thought broadcasting
   (d)   Thought insertion with dysphasia
   (e)   Thought withdrawal with pressured speech

Derailment refers to a breakdown in association of thoughts so that there seems to be no understandable connection between them. It is a severe form of thought disorder that indicates the patient is very unwell. Neologisms are 'new' invented words, which can have meaning for the patient, but might not be understandable to the observer. Neologisms can occur alongside any thought disorder. See Oyebode (2008).

6   A 34-year-old man believes that his neighbours are trying to force him to leave his property. He believes they are sending threatening messages in Morse code through the radiators in his apartment. He also believes they are taunting him by having a small English flag on their car during the World Cup, as he is originally from Poland. He is adamant that he is correct despite you offering alternative and more likely explanations. How would you classify the nature of his beliefs?

   (a)   **Persecutory delusions**
   (b)   Grandiose delusions
   (c)   Delusions of control
   (d)   Over-valued ideas
   (e)   Thought insertion

This is an example of a set of persecutory delusions, the most frequent type of delusion. These can arise in many different conditions, including severe depression, mania and delirium, as well as schizophrenia. The patient's response to the beliefs can vary – in schizophrenia, the affect can sometimes be blunted or inappropriately indifferent (an 'incongruent affect'). It is clear this man's beliefs are delusional rather than over-valued ideas as they are held with unusual conviction and not amenable to logic. See Oyebode (2008).

7 A 54-year-old woman with a history of bipolar disorder complains that nursing staff on the ward are interfering with her 'special mission' to rid the city of sin. She says she should be allowed to leave the ward and continue her good work. She says she knows she has been chosen by God to do this work as when she prays, she feels 'full of energy and love'. Her husband tells you that although she attends church regularly, these beliefs are new and out of character for her. How would you describe her beliefs?

    (a)   Nihilistic delusions
    (b)   Delusions of prayer
    (c)   Delusions of power
    (d)   Over-valued ideas
    (e)   **Religious delusions**

Religious delusions are common. They can be grandiose in nature, as is the case here. That a religious belief might seem bizarre to the observer, however, does not make it delusional. Professor Andrew Sims has written authoritatively on the subject and states 'Religious delusions are not caused by excessive religious belief, nor by the wrongdoing which the patient might attribute as cause, but they simply accentuate that when a person becomes mentally ill his delusions reflect, in their content, his predominant interests and concerns'. See Sims (2012).

8 A 23-year-old man believes that his bowels are being twisted by an alien force that originated on Mars but now lives in Malta. What feature of this delusion makes it more likely that his diagnosis is schizophrenia?

    (a)   It involves aliens
    (b)   It involves Malta
    (c)   **It is bizarre**
    (d)   It is a primary delusion
    (e)   It involves his bowels

Bizarre delusions are considered important in psychiatry. They are thought to be more indicative of schizophrenia than other types of delusion and their presence was previously considered a sufficient criterion to make a diagnosis of schizophrenia, so long as dysfunction/suffering and length-of-illness criteria were satisfied. Cermolacce *et al* (2010) called into question the validity of 'bizarreness', and it is no longer considered a sufficient criterion for a diagnosis of schizophrenia.

There is a long history of attempts to define a bizarre delusion. Emil Kraepelin defined delusions in schizophrenia as 'nonsensical', and Karl Jaspers considered them 'incomprehensible'. Kindler conceived the bizarreness of a delusion on a spectrum, whereas Sims stressed that the 'un-understandable' component of a delusion is central to it being a primary delusion, rather than indicative of diagnosis per se. See Oyebode (2008).

9 A 43-year-old father of three believes his wife is having an affair. He has been examining her laundry and trying to access her email account. There is no basis in reality to his belief and he has no proof to support it. However, he is adamant that he is correct. His wife has tried to reassure him but she feels this is just making it worse. What is this man's diagnosis?

   (a) Delusion of love
   (b) **Morbid jealousy**
   (c) Sexual envy disorder
   (d) Delusion of control
   (e) Erotomania

Morbid jealousy is a specific disorder of the content of thought. Here, the patient unreasonably believes his or her partner is being sexually unfaithful. The form can vary: if the belief is held to delusional intensity, it can be referred to as a 'delusion of infidelity'. It might be an isolated symptom (a delusional disorder), but more commonly occurs as part of schizophrenia. However, morbid jealousy can be conceived as existing on a spectrum and can also occur in the form of an over-valued idea or obsessional belief.

In the majority of cases, there is no basis in reality for the belief. However, it can be argued that delusions of infidelity can still be pathological even where a partner is unfaithful, when there is no logical evidence being adduced for the beliefs. German psychiatrist Karl Jaspers (see further reading) introduced the important concept that delusions should be diagnosed on the basis of their form (the way in which the belief is held) rather than of their content (the belief itself). The patient might go to extreme lengths to find proof and there is a significant risk of violence. Morbid jealousy more commonly affects men than women and is associated with alcohol and substance misuse. See Kingham & Gordon (2004) and Oyebode (2008) and, for further reading, Oyebode (2013).

10 A 65-year-old woman tells you at the out-patient clinic that her husband has been replaced by a double. This person looks the same as her husband and shares the same mannerisms as him, but in her view is certainly not her husband. How would you describe her beliefs?

   (a) Folie à deux
   (b) Delusional infidelity
   (c) Delusional interpretation
   (d) **Capgras syndrome**
   (e) Delusional memory

This woman is exhibiting Capgras syndrome, a form of delusional misidentification. It is a rare disorder in which the person believes that another person, usually closely related to them, has been replaced by an exact double. Capgras syndrome is similar to the other misidentification syndromes: intermetamorphosis (believing a person has been transformed into a different person), Fregoli syndrome (believing a stranger is someone familiar) and the syndrome of subjective doubles (believing that another person has been transformed into your own self). See Oyebode (2008).

11 A 57-year-old man believes the electricity company is persecuting him by sending error messages on a website and by making the lights flicker on and off at night. As there is no evidence, his wife initially does not believe him, but over time comes to share his belief. What is this phenomenon called?

(a) **Folie à deux**
(b) Delusions of control
(c) Delusional interpretation
(d) Delusions of infestation
(e) Fregoli syndrome

Folie à deux is an uncommon occurrence, whereby a delusional belief is transferred from a psychotic person to another individual, usually someone in close proximity to them. The associate is usually socially, intellectually or physically deprived or disadvantaged. See Oyebode (2008) and, for further reading, Shimizu *et al* (2007).

12 A 33-year-old woman with paranoid schizophrenia describes hearing voices when there is no one around. They are both male and female and they tell her to harm others. She finds them very distressing and it is difficult for her to resist acting on them. How would you describe this symptom?

(a) Sensory distortion
(b) Third-person auditory hallucination
(c) **Second-person command auditory hallucination**
(d) Pseudohallucination
(e) Autoscopic hallucination

This patient's hallucination is auditory, as it occurs in the form of voices. It can be described as second-person (because the voices speak directly to her) and also as command (because they give her orders). There are many ways to define hallucinations, the most straightforward being 'a perception without an object'. Hallucination differs from sensory distortion (variation in the intensity, quality or associated feeling of a perception) and illusion (misinterpretations of real stimuli). Hallucination can occur in any sensory modality, but auditory hallucination is the most common form in psychosis, with prevalence estimates of up to 72% in people with schizophrenia. Research in the past two decades indicates it is not uncommon in the general population also.

Command hallucination is an example of a 'threat–control override' symptom. Many clinicians believe such symptoms to be associated with increased violence. There is considerable debate about the validity of this concept, however. See Oyebode (2008) and, for further reading, Mueser *et al* (1990), Linscott & van Os (2013) and Stompe *et al* (2004).

13

13 A 23-year-old man describes hearing voices inside his head, talking about him. They say things like 'I think he should harm himself' and also argue between themselves. He cannot dismiss the voices at will. The voices seem real. How would you describe this symptom?

    (a)   Pseudohallucination
    (b)   **Third-person auditory hallucination**
    (c)   Running commentary
    (d)   Sensory distortion
    (e)   Illusion

This man is experiencing a third-person auditory hallucination – a first-rank symptom of schizophrenia – in the form of voices heard arguing or discussing. They have a real quality and are difficult to dismiss.

The patient describes the voices as occurring inside his head, and this might lead some readers to think this represents a pseudohallucination. The qualities of pseudohallucination, as traditionally conceived in psychiatry, have been described well by Sims. However, a strong note of caution is advised in using this term, which seems to lack clinical validity. See Oyebode (2008) and, for further reading, Van der Zwaard & Polak (2001).

14 A 19-year-old college student who has been drinking and taking drugs regularly for several weeks is admitted to hospital feeling unwell. Within a day, he develops the sensation of insects crawling inside his skin. There is no evidence that there are insects there. What is the correct term for his symptom?

    (a)   Olfactory hallucination
    (b)   Visual hallucination
    (c)   Auditory hallucination
    (d)   Gustatory hallucination
    (e)   **Formication**

Formication is a particularly unpleasant form of haptic or tactile hallucination, associated with intoxication or withdrawal from alcohol and drugs, particularly cocaine. It can also occur in psychosis, as can hallucination in other sensory modalities: taste (gustatory), smell (olfactory) and vision (visual). See Oyebode (2008).

15 A 68-year-old man has cognitive impairment and Parkinsonism, but no history of schizophrenia. He complains of seeing spiders in his room during the day over the course of several weeks. He describes them in great detail and seems frightened of them. There is no evidence that there are spiders in his room. What do you think is the most likely cause for this symptom?

    (a)   Old age
    (b)   **Dementia with Lewy bodies**
    (c)   Schizophrenia
    (d)   Alzheimer's disease
    (e)   Depression

This man probably has dementia with Lewy bodies. He has cognitive decline (a central feature) as well as the other two core features: visual hallucination and Parkinsonism. It is very important to note that, although visual hallucination can occur in psychosis, it is much more common in organic illness and should prompt the treating doctor to look for an organic cause.

Onset of psychosis can occur in older age, but is very uncommon. Visual hallucination can occur in Alzheimer's disease, but the overall clinical picture here is more in keeping with dementia with Lewy bodies. See McKeith *et al* (2004).

16 A 72-year-old woman is asked to immediately repeat back three words that are said to her in the MMSE. What component of memory does this test?

   (a)   Short-term memory
   (b)   Recall
   (c)   Medium-term memory
   (d)   Long-term memory
   (e)   **Registration**

What is commonly referred to as 'memory' consists of an interplay between many different components, such as registration of information, storage of information, recognition of information (that one has encountered the fact/image/smell before) and recollection of information at a chosen moment. Asking a patient repeat words back tests only registration: the receiving, processing and combining of received information. It does not require the patient to remember the information for any length of time, simply to demonstrate that they registered it. Registration may be impaired by attentional deficits.

A further classification distinguishes between declarative memory (which can be autobiographical or semantic/factual) and implicit memory (such as how to ride a bike or write). Using the terms 'short' and 'long' to refer to memory can be confusing and is often unhelpful clinically. Most use of the term 'short-term memory' refers to 'working memory' as described by Baddeley: the temporary storage and manipulation of information that is assumed to be necessary for a wide range of complex cognitive activities. See Oyebode (2008) and, for further reading, Baddeley (2003).

17 A consultant asks one of her patients, who has a diagnosis of schizophrenia, whether or not the patient believes he has an illness. She asks him if he needs medication and if he needs to stay in hospital. What part of the mental state examination is this?

    (a)   Memory tests
    (b)   Investigation of knowledge
    (c)   Test of attention
    (d)   **Investigating insight**
    (e)   Developing rapport

Lack of insight is a common feature of schizophrenia. It is associated with non-compliance with medication and poor outcomes for patients. Insight is multi-dimensional and is not a binary concept; insight into different aspects of one's illness and life occur on a spectrum. Insight has been the focus of a considerable amount of research. See Oyebode (2008) and, for further reading, Buckley *et al* (2007) and Mintz *et al* (2003).

EMI answers

Thought disorder

Options:

    (a)   Flight of ideas
    (b)   Thought block
    (c)   Derailment
    (d)   Tangentiality
    (e)   Thought insertion
    (f)   Circumstantiality
    (g)   Thought withdrawal
    (h)   Thought broadcasting

From the list above, select the correct symptom for each of the scenarios below.

1 A 35-year-old man with schizophrenia is speaking very quickly and jumps from subject to subject. There seems to be no connection between his thoughts and what he says does not make any sense to you.

(c) Derailment

2 A 28-year-old woman with bipolar disorder in conversation and does not get back to her original topic.

(d) Tangentiality

3 A 56-year-old woman with delirium develops depressive psychosis. She believes the nursing staff are 'stealing' thoughts from her head using equipment in her hospital room.

(g) Thought withdrawal

Types of delusion

Options:

- (a) Delusions of grandeur
- (b) Delusions of infestation
- (c) Persecutory delusions
- (d) Capgras syndrome
- (e) Delusions of infidelity
- (f) Folie à deux
- (g) Nihilistic delusions
- (h) Erotomania

From the list above, select the correct term for each of the delusions below.

1 A 22-year-old man believes the police are watching him on camera. He thinks they are doing this as they have an agenda to harm him and send him to prison. There is no evidence that this is the case.

(c) Persecutory delusions

2 A 48-year-old man has a long-standing belief that he is infected with lice. He cannot see or feel the lice but he says he 'just know[s] they are there'. There is no evidence this is the case. He persists in this belief despite being otherwise well.

(b) Delusions of infestation

3 A 20-year-old woman believes that a Member of Parliament (whom she has never met) is in love with her. She believes she has to be with him or her life will be over and goes to extreme lengths to make this happen.

(h) Erotomania

Memory problems

Options:

- (a) Working memory
- (b) Semantic memory
- (c) Implicit memory
- (d) Registration deficit
- (e) Confabulation
- (f) Declarative memory
- (g) Recall deficit
- (h) Anterograde memory loss
- (i) Autobiographical memory

From the list above, select the area of deficit and/or type of deficit for each of the cases below. (There is more than one correct answer for some of the scenarios.)

1 A 72-year-old man only remembers one of the three items read to him on the MMSE, although he was able to repeat them back to you initially.

(g) Recall deficit

2 A 54-year-old man who has been involved in a road traffic accident has a memory deficit for what happened for 24 h after the event

(h) Anterograde memory loss

3   An 85-year-old woman with advanced Alzheimer's disease cannot recall many details from the last few years of her life or the name of the current Prime Minister.

   (b) Semantic memory

   (i) Autobiographical memory

4   A 35-year-old athlete who had a head injury struggles on tests of cognitive performance. When asked about recent events he cannot recall, he 'fills in the gaps', giving false information.

   (e) Confabulation

CHAPTER 2

Psychotic disorders

MCQs

1   A 22-year-old man presents with a 2-month history of third-person auditory hallucinations, thought broadcasting and persecutory delusions. No other symptoms are described. He has a history of depression, for which he received antidepressant therapy at the age of 20. He used cannabinoids on a weekly basis from the age of 17 to 21, but hasn't used them for the past 4 months. What is the most likely diagnosis?

    (a)   Paranoid schizophrenia
    (b)   Schizoaffective disorder, depressive type
    (c)   Drug-induced psychosis
    (d)   Delusional disorder
    (e)   Acute psychotic disorder

2   A young man has recently been diagnosed with paranoid schizophrenia. He is attending the clinic today and is anxious to learn more about the diagnosis and wishes to discuss symptoms that he might experience as part of the disorder. All the following are negative symptoms of schizophrenia, except:

    (a)   Affective flattening
    (b)   Avolition
    (c)   Anhedonia
    (d)   Asociality
    (e)   Aggressiveness

3   A person who had one episode of hypomania and six episodes of depression meets the diagnostic criteria for which one of the following?

    (a)   Recurrent depressive disorder
    (b)   Cyclothymia
    (c)   Bipolar affective disorder
    (d)   Dysthymia
    (e)   Schizoaffective disorder

4   You are called to assess a 24-year-old woman who gave birth 3 days ago. She has been behaving bizarrely on the obstetrics ward, accusing staff of spying on her and of harming her baby. She hasn't slept for 24 h and is displaying overactivity and aggression. You assess the woman and diagnose a psychotic episode. All the following are risk factors for a postpartum psychosis, except:

   (a)   Primiparity
   (b)   Bipolar affective disorder
   (c)   Obstetric complications
   (d)   Gender of child
   (e)   Single marital status

5   In bipolar affective disorder, which one of the following is correct?

   (a)   It usually presents with delusions of control on mental state exam
   (b)   Hypermania is a severe form of mania
   (c)   Depressive mood swings are usually accompanied by psychotic symptoms
   (d)   Manic episodes are often associated with irritability rather than elevated mood
   (e)   At least three episodes of mania are required for its diagnosis

6   A 22-year-old woman presents to the clinic after a referral by her GP. Her mood is currently euthymic, but she reports three episodes of brief mood elation over the past 3 months, without significant functional impairment. She was previously treated for a depressive episode at the age of 19. She is concerned that she might have bipolar affective disorder. What duration of mood elation would be required to allow for a hypomanic episode to be diagnosed?

   (a)   At least 1 day
   (b)   At least 4 days
   (c)   At least 1 week
   (d)   At least 2 weeks
   (e)   At least 1 month

7   A 30-year-old man has been diagnosed with bipolar affective disorder after experiencing a second episode of mania with psychotic features. He was hospitalised for a period of 3 months and was euthymic when discharged on mood-stabilising medication to prevent a manic relapse. Which of the following medications is the least effective protection against relapse of mania?

   (a)   Lithium carbonate
   (b)   Sodium valproate
   (c)   Carbamazepine
   (d)   Lamotrigine
   (e)   Olanzapine

8   A 25-year-old woman is admitted to hospital with a diagnosis of mania with psychotic symptoms. She presented with a 2-week history of mood elation, decreased sleep, overactivity, impulsive behaviour, racing thoughts, grandiose delusions, and reported hearing voices commenting on her actions. Schneiderian first-rank symptoms are reported to occur at what frequency in manic psychosis?

(a)   1–5%
(b)   10–20%
(c)   30–40%
(d)   50–60%
(e)   80–90%

9   A 20-year-old man is brought to the clinic accompanied by his mother. He has a 10-day history of irritable mood, which is abnormal for him and has prevented him functioning in his normal occupational and social activities. He has been restless and overactive, with social disinhibition and grandiose delusions evident. Which of the following statements regarding manic episodes is false?

(a)   They are characterised by severe elevations of mood or irritability
(b)   The majority of patients with mania will have psychotic symptoms at some point in their illness
(c)   The patient will generally be able to maintain an adequate level of functioning
(d)   They can be precipitated by antidepressant therapy
(e)   Symptoms can be mimicked by frontal-lobe pathology

10 A 23-year-old man has been recently diagnosed with paranoid schizophrenia. He is attending the clinic accompanied by his mother. She wishes to ask about known risk factors that might predict the development of paranoid schizophrenia. The following are risk factors for the development of paranoid schizophrenia, except:

(a)   Poor parenting
(b)   Being an immigrant
(c)   Obstetric complications
(d)   Urban living
(e)   Family history of psychotic illness

11 The father of a 26-year-old woman recently diagnosed with paranoid schizophrenia wishes to discuss with you his daughter's prognosis. Which of the following factors in her history might be considered a poor prognostic factor for recovery?

(a)   Adult onset
(b)   Married at onset
(c)   Insidious onset
(d)   Less socially disadvantaged at onset
(e)   Mood symptoms at onset

12 A local GP wishes to discuss with you the large number of young adults with psychosis she has seen in her surgery of late. You both work in a city with a population of 100 000. You plan to discuss with her the epidemiology of psychotic disorders, in particular schizophrenia. What is the expected incidence of schizophrenia in this population?

(a) 1/100 000
(b) 5/100 000
(c) 15/100 000
(d) 50/100 000
(e) 100/100 000

13 A 23-year-old man is attending the clinic, having recently been diagnosed with first-episode psychosis. He is currently receiving treatment and is stable. Which of the following risk factors would be most predictive of a psychotic relapse for this patient?

(a) Premorbid social isolation
(b) Medication adherence
(c) Abstinence from alcohol use
(d) Low expressed emotion in his family
(e) Continuing education

14 A 65-year-old man is referred to the clinic by his GP. For the past year he has believed that his neighbours have been conspiring against him. He believes that they plan to harm him and feels threatened by them. Prior to the onset of this belief, he had been good friends with his neighbours and collateral history indicates that he has nothing to fear from them. Besides the presence of this delusional belief, his mental state examination is unremarkable. What is the probable diagnosis?

(a) Alzheimer's disease
(b) Paranoid schizophrenia
(c) Severe depression with psychotic symptoms
(d) Paranoid personality disorder
(e) Delusional disorder

15 You are called to the emergency department to review a 25-year-old man. He was brought to the emergency department by ambulance after being found unconscious in his front garden. He had taken an overdose of codeine and benzodiazepines in response to second-person command hallucinations and claims that he is no longer able to resist their instructions. He has had no previous contact with psychiatric services. He is now medically stable. What is the most appropriate management intervention?

   (a) Recommend treatment with antipsychotic medication and discharge for out-patient follow-up over the next week
   (b) Arrange for the patient to be followed up at home in the coming days by the community mental health team
   (c) Admit to the medical ward of the hospital
   (d) Admission to the psychiatric unit of the hospital
   (e) Recommend treatment with an SSRI and discharge for out-patient follow-up over the next week

16 A 25-year-old man presents to the clinic with a 1-year history of functional decline and psychotic symptoms. He presents with third-person auditory hallucinations that give a running commentary on his thoughts and actions, bizarre delusions, including believing that he is the father of the Queen of England, and describes thought withdrawal. He displays formal thought disorder, with derailment and neologisms prominent. He has experienced recurrent episodes of mood disturbance for extended periods over the past 2 years and currently displays features of mania. He intermittently uses cannabis and previously used amphetamines, but stopped 6 months ago. What is the probable diagnosis?

   (a) Paranoid schizophrenia
   (b) Drug-induced psychosis
   (c) Delusional disorder
   (d) Schizoaffective disorder
   (e) Bipolar affective disorder

17 A 26-year-old woman has been diagnosed with a first episode of paranoid schizophrenia. Which of the following is the most appropriate treatment option?

   (a) Flupentixol decanoate
   (b) Olanzapine
   (c) Fluoxetine
   (d) Diazepam
   (e) Lithium carbonate

18 A 27-year-old man was reviewed at the clinic by the consultant psychiatrist with you in attendance. The consultant psychiatrist informed you that the patient had a diagnosis of treatment-resistant schizophrenia. What is a recognised diagnostic criterion for treatment-resistant schizophrenia?

(a) No antipsychotic medication is effective
(b) Only injectable antipsychotic medication is effective
(c) Lack of clinical response to trials of two different low-dose antipsychotics
(d) Lack of clinical response to two different antipsychotics at optimal dose and for sufficient duration
(e) Lack of clinical response to antipsychotic medication because of comorbid affective disorder

19 A 26-year-old man attends the clinic with a history of unremitting psychotic symptoms since the onset of his illness 1 year ago. He has been treated with three different antipsychotics, olanzapine (20 mg daily), risperidone (6 mg daily) and haloperidol (15 mg daily), without achieving a therapeutic response. The consultant on the team asks you to review the patient's presentation and history to exclude comorbid features that might be leading to the treatment resistance/non-response. All the following can impact on antipsychotic treatment response, except:

(a) Marital status
(b) Comorbid depression
(c) Alcohol misuse
(d) Medication non-adherence
(e) Recurring stressor

20 A 25-year-old woman attends the early intervention service for the treatment of first-episode psychosis. All the following are recommended interventions in first-episode psychosis, except:

(a) Cognitive–behavioural therapy
(b) Family involvement and support
(c) High-dose antipsychotic medication
(d) Educational and vocational rehabilitation
(e) Relapse prevention strategy

EMI questions

Diagnosis

Options:

    (a)   Paranoid schizophrenia
    (b)   Delusional disorder, somatic type
    (c)   Manic episode with mood-congruent psychotic features
    (d)   Delusional misidentification
    (e)   Schizoaffective disorder
    (f)   Substance-induced psychotic disorder
    (g)   Delusional disorder, persecutory type
    (h)   Severe depressive episode with mood-congruent psychotic features

For each of the following clinical vignettes, please select the probable diagnosis.

1   A 25-year-old man complains that he is being spied on by the intelligence services. He reports that his house is bugged and that he can hear agents speaking about what he is doing. He is convinced that this is happening and states that it started 6 months ago.

2   A 64-year-old woman presents to her GP with multiple physical complaints. She reports that she has felt tired and exhausted for the past few months. She tells her GP that her 'body is dead' and that she can hear her dead husband calling her to join him.

3   A 22-year-old woman presents to the emergency department, reporting that her college classmates wish to kill her. She is highly distressed and agitated. She became acutely aware of this threat to her safety 2 days previously and reports that, since then, she has been hiding in her bedroom with a knife to protect herself. She reports that she has heard the voices of her classmates discussing her and laughing about her. She had used amphetamines 4 days ago.

Treatment choices

Options:

    (a)   Stop clozapine
    (b)   Start hyoscine hydrobromide
    (c)   Reduce clozapine
    (d)   Add antidepressant
    (e)   Start depot medication
    (f)   Increase clozapine
    (g)   Admit to hospital
    (h)   Add amisulpride

Select an intervention that would be recommended for each of the following clinical scenarios.

1 A 33-year-old woman, treated with clozapine in the community, presents reporting reduced energy over the past month. She reports feeling low, has lost interest in day-to-day activities, is sleeping poorly and reports poor concentration.

2 A 28-year-old man is being titrated with clozapine. He complains that his pillow is soaking wet when he wakes in the morning.

3 A 30-year-old man has been treated with clozapine for 6 months. He reports that he stopped smoking cigarettes 2 weeks ago. Today he seems sedated and reports that he has been constipated over the past week.

Treatment choices

Options:
- (a) Quetiapine
- (b) Depot medication
- (c) Electroconvulsive therapy
- (d) Lamotrigine
- (e) Clozapine
- (f) Antidepressant medication
- (g) Hospital admission
- (h) Lithium carbonate

Select an intervention that would be recommended for each of the following clinical scenarios.

1 A 26-year-old woman with a diagnosis of schizophrenia is admitted to hospital following a relapse of psychosis. This is her third hospitalisation in the past year and all have occurred secondary to non-adherence to oral antipsychotic medication. She had previously responded to oral antipsychotic medication when adherent.

2 A 34-year-old man with a diagnosis of schizophrenia presents to A&E reporting command hallucinations and suicidal thoughts.

3 A 28-year-old man with a history of schizophrenia presents to the clinic with ongoing psychotic symptoms, having failed to respond to three different antipsychotic treatments.

MCQ answers

1   A 22-year-old man presents with a 2-month history of third-person auditory
    hallucinations, thought broadcasting and persecutory delusions. No other symptoms
    are described. He has a history of depression, for which he received antidepressant
    therapy at the age of 20. He used cannabinoids on a weekly basis from the age of 17
    to 21, but hasn't used them for the past 4 months. What is the most likely diagnosis?

    (a)   **Paranoid schizophrenia**
    (b)   Schizoaffective disorder, depressive type
    (c)   Drug-induced psychosis
    (d)   Delusional disorder
    (e)   Acute psychotic disorder

This patient meets the ICD-10 diagnostic criteria for paranoid schizophrenia,
presenting with psychotic symptoms of > 1 month's duration. The duration
of symptoms rules out an acute psychotic disorder. The nature of the
symptoms and the lack of recent drug use exclude drug-induced psychosis.
Although individuals with delusional disorder can experience transient
auditory hallucinations, the presence of third-person auditory hallucinations
and thought broadcasting – first-rank symptoms – are strongly suggestive of
paranoid schizophrenia. Illness duration must be > 3 months for delusional
disorder to be diagnosed using ICD-10 diagnostic criteria. The patient has
had one prior episode of depression and there is no history of psychotic
symptoms occurring concurrent to mood disturbance, making a diagnosis
of schizoaffective disorder unlikely at this stage. See WHO (1992).

2   A young man has recently been diagnosed with paranoid schizophrenia. He is
    attending the clinic today and is anxious to learn more about the diagnosis and wishes
    to discuss symptoms that he might experience as part of the disorder. All the following
    are negative symptoms of schizophrenia, except:

    (a)   Affective flattening
    (b)   Avolition
    (c)   Anhedonia
    (d)   Asociality
    (e)   **Aggressiveness**

The negative symptom construct includes blunted/flat affect, anhedonia
(diminished interest and enjoyment), alogia (poverty of speech), asociality
(social withdrawal) and avolition (diminished motivation and initiative).
It is important to assess for the cause of negative symptoms and to exclude
comorbid factors that might be causing the symptoms. Primary negative
symptoms occur as part of the schizophrenia disorder, whereas secondary
negative symptoms can be caused by positive psychotic symptoms,
depression, or extrapyramidal side-effects.

A pathophysiologically distinct negative syndrome has been recognised
within schizophrenia. This syndrome is known as a deficit syndrome and
is diagnosed on the basis of the presence of primary enduring negative
symptoms over at least 12 months. See Buchanan (2007).

3   A person who had one episode of hypomania and six episodes of depression meets the diagnostic criteria for which one of the following?

    (a)   Recurrent depressive disorder
    (b)   Cyclothymia
    (c)   **Bipolar affective disorder**
    (d)   Dysthymia
    (e)   Schizoaffective disorder

The ICD-10 diagnostic criteria for bipolar affective disorder require two discrete mood episodes, at least one of which must be a hypomanic/manic episode. In DSM-5, a single episode of mania or a single episode of hypomania plus a single major depressive episode is sufficient to diagnose bipolar affective disorder. See APA (2013) and WHO (1992).

4   You are called to assess a 24-year-old woman who gave birth 3 days ago. She has been behaving bizarrely on the obstetrics ward, accusing staff of spying on her and of harming her baby. She hasn't slept for 24 h and is displaying overactivity and aggression. You assess the woman and diagnose a psychotic episode. All the following are risk factors for a postpartum psychosis, except:

    (a)   Primiparity
    (b)   Bipolar affective disorder
    (c)   Obstetric complications
    (d)   **Gender of child**
    (e)   Single marital status

Postpartum psychosis is strongly related to bipolar affective disorder. Postpartum psychosis is the most uncommon, but most severe, form of postnatal affective illness, with rates of 1–2 episodes per 1000 deliveries. Postpartum psychosis is generally rapid in onset and can begin within 24–72 h of the birth, with the majority of episodes occurring within 2 weeks of the birth. It is hallmarked by mood disturbance (either elation or depression), disorganised behaviour, delusions and hallucinations. It is a psychiatric emergency and generally necessitates hospitalisation for treatment. Risk factors for its occurrence include: a personal history of bipolar affective disorder or postpartum psychosis, a family history of postpartum psychosis or bipolar affective disorder, being single, primiparity (first birth) and obstetric complications. See Jones & Smith (2009) and Kendell *et al* (1987).

5   In bipolar affective disorder, which one of the following is correct?

    (a)   It usually presents with delusions of control on mental state exam
    (b)   Hypermania is a severe form of mania
    (c)   Depressive mood swings are usually accompanied by psychotic symptoms
    (d)   **Manic episodes are often associated with irritability rather than elevated mood**
    (e)   At least three episodes of mania are required for its diagnosis

The key feature of bipolar affective disorder is the experience of recurrent episodes of hypomania or mania – grandiose and expansive affect associated with increased drive and decreased sleep, with the mood being elated, expansive or irritable – and recurrent depressive episodes. All the features reported in mania, except psychotic symptoms, can also occur in hypomania to a less severe extent. Hypermania does not exist as a descriptive term for mania. See WHO (1992).

6   A 22-year-old woman presents to the clinic after a referral by her GP. Her mood is currently euthymic, but she reports three episodes of brief mood elation over the past 3 months, without significant functional impairment. She was previously treated for a depressive episode at the age of 19. She is concerned that she might have bipolar affective disorder. What duration of mood elation would be required to allow for a hypomanic episode to be diagnosed?

(a)   At least 1 day
(b)   **At least 4 days**
(c)   At least 1 week
(d)   At least 2 weeks
(e)   At least 1 month

According to ICD-10 and DSM-5 diagnostic criteria, mood elation/ irritability must last at least 4 days to qualify for the diagnosis of a hypomanic episode. However, there is considerable debate among clinicians about how long hypomanic symptoms should be present for to make a diagnosis of hypomania: many clinicians assert that some individuals have periods of mood elation lasting for less than 4 days. In hypomania, all the features reported in mania, except psychotic symptoms, can also occur but to a lesser extent. The patient with hypomania will not experience severe social or occupational functional impairment. They might view their increased productivity as a positive experience, although the changes in their behaviour might be noted by others who know them. See Saunders & Goodwin (2010) and WHO (1992).

7   A 30-year-old man has been diagnosed with bipolar affective disorder after experiencing a second episode of mania with psychotic features. He was hospitalised for a period of 3 months and was euthymic when discharged on mood-stabilising medication to prevent a manic relapse. Which of the following medications is the least effective protection against relapse of mania?

(a)   Lithium carbonate
(b)   Sodium valproate
(c)   Carbamazepine
(d)   **Lamotrigine**
(e)   Olanzapine

All these medications are licensed as mood stabilisers in bipolar affective disorder. However, lamotrigine is not effective for the prevention of manic relapse and is not recommended as maintenance treatment for mania prophylaxis. Lamotrigine prevents depressive relapses more than manic relapses. If a patient's illness course is predominantly one of manic relapse, maintenance treatment will require the use of a more effective manic prophylaxis, such as lithium carbonate, olanzapine, sodium valproate or carbamazepine. See Taylor *et al* (2012).

8   A 25-year-old woman is admitted to hospital with a diagnosis of mania with psychotic symptoms. She presented with a 2-week history of mood elation, decreased sleep, overactivity, impulsive behaviour, racing thoughts, grandiose delusions, and reported hearing voices commenting on her actions. Schneiderian first-rank symptoms are reported to occur at what frequency in manic psychosis?

   (a)   1–5%
   (b)   **10–20%**
   (c)   30–40%
   (d)   50–60%
   (e)   80–90%

Mania with psychotic symptoms is most commonly associated with grandiose delusions and mood-congruent auditory hallucinations: for example, the voice of a famous person telling you that you are destined for greatness. Persecutory delusions can develop, emerging when an individual believes that others are thwarting their grandiose plans.

One of the most prominent models for schizophrenia has been the concept of first-rank symptoms (see question 1 in Chapter 1). First-rank symptoms are present in 57–88% of individuals with schizophrenia, but are not specific to schizophrenia. They have been reported to occur in 10–20% of manic episodes. See Nordgaard *et al* (2008).

9   A 20-year-old man is brought to the clinic accompanied by his mother. He has a 10-day history of irritable mood, which is abnormal for him and has prevented him functioning in his normal occupational and social activities. He has been restless and overactive, with social disinhibition and grandiose delusions evident. Which of the following statements regarding manic episodes is false?

   (a)   They are characterised by severe elevations of mood or irritability
   (b)   The majority of patients with mania will have psychotic symptoms at some point in their illness
   (c)   **The patient will generally be able to maintain an adequate level of functioning**
   (d)   They can be precipitated by antidepressant therapy
   (e)   Symptoms can be mimicked by frontal-lobe pathology

In the ICD-10 diagnostic criteria for 'mania without psychotic symptoms', mood is elevated, out of keeping with the patient's circumstances and can vary from carefree joviality to almost uncontrollable excitement. Elation is accompanied by increased energy, resulting in overactivity, pressure of speech and a decreased need for sleep. Attention cannot be sustained and there is often marked distractibility. Self-esteem is often inflated, with grandiose ideas and over-confidence. Loss of normal social inhibitions might result in behaviour that is reckless, foolhardy or inappropriate to the circumstances and out of character.

Mania is associated with a decline in an individual's level of educational, occupational and social functioning; at times the behaviour exhibited during a manic episode can be a source of considerable embarrassment for the individual on recovery from the mania. Loss of insight can occur during mania and often mania requires hospitalisation for treatment, in comparison to hypomania, which is generally treated in an out-patient setting. See WHO (1992).

10 A 23-year-old man has been recently diagnosed with paranoid schizophrenia. He is attending the clinic accompanied by his mother. She wishes to ask about known risk factors that might predict the development of paranoid schizophrenia. The following are risk factors for the development of paranoid schizophrenia, except:

(a) **Poor parenting**
(b) Being an immigrant
(c) Obstetric complications
(d) Urban living
(e) Family history of psychotic illness

Childhood adversity, such as the loss of a parent or abuse, is a risk factor for schizophrenia; however, poor parenting is not. Schizophrenia is highly heritable: having one parent with schizophrenia increases the risk of the child developing the disorder to 10–15%, and having both parents with schizophrenia increases the risk to 40%. Being an immigrant is associated with a relative risk of schizophrenia of 2.9, and having grown up in a city is also associated with increased risk of developing schizophrenia. See Howes & Murray (2014).

11 The father of a 26-year-old woman recently diagnosed with paranoid schizophrenia wishes to discuss with you his daughter's prognosis. Which of the following factors in her history might be considered a poor prognostic factor for recovery?

(a) Adult onset
(b) Married at onset
(c) **Insidious onset**
(d) Less socially disadvantaged at onset
(e) Mood symptoms at onset

Longitudinal follow-up studies of patients diagnosed with schizophrenia have found that 15–40% achieve social or functional recovery. Factors associated with an improved prognosis include: mood symptoms at illness onset; improved social integration at onset; and less social disadvantage at onset. An insidious onset, characterised by longer duration of untreated psychosis, is associated with a worse prognosis and lower rates of recovery, as are early age at onset and greater severity of cognitive and negative symptoms. See Jaaskelainen *et al* (2013) and Lieberman *et al* (1996).

12 A local GP wishes to discuss with you the large number of young adults with psychosis she has seen in her surgery of late. You both work in a city with a population of 100 000. You plan to discuss with her the epidemiology of psychotic disorders, in particular schizophrenia. What is the expected incidence of schizophrenia in this population?

  (a) 1/100 000
  (b) 5/100 000
  (c) **15/100 000**
  (d) 50/100 000
  (e) 100/100 000

The distribution of a disease is generally expressed in terms of incidence (new cases), and prevalence (total number of cases: existing plus new). Incidence refers to the number of new cases of the disease that develop over a specific period of time among people who are at risk for developing the disease.

The incidence of schizophrenia in the UK and USA is approximately 15/100 000, meaning that 15 new cases of schizophrenia per 100 000 of the population develop in each calendar year. Estimates of the risk of developing schizophrenia over one's lifetime range between 0.3% and 2.0%, with an average of approximately 0.7–1.0%. See McGrath *et al* (2008).

13 A 23-year-old man is attending the clinic, having recently been diagnosed with first-episode psychosis. He is currently receiving treatment and is stable. Which of the following risk factors would be most predictive of a psychotic relapse for this patient?

  (a) **Premorbid social isolation**
  (b) Medication adherence
  (c) Abstinence from alcohol use
  (d) Low expressed emotion in his family
  (e) Continuing education

Factors associated with relapse in first-episode psychosis and the early stages of a psychotic illness include the following: Poor treatment engagement; alcohol/substance use disorder; high expressed emotion in family setting; poor premorbid social functioning; increased severity of cognitive symptoms. Medication adherence would not predispose to relapse, but medication non-adherence (also known as non-compliance) would do so.

Expressed emotion is a construct that seeks to capture the emotional environment within a patient's family. High levels of expressed emotion robustly predict higher relapse rates. There are five components to expressed emotion: emotional over-involvement, critical comments, hostility, positive remarks and warmth. See Bhugra & McKenzie (2003).

14 A 65-year-old man is referred to the clinic by his GP. For the past year he has believed
that his neighbours have been conspiring against him. He believes that they plan to
harm him and feels threatened by them. Prior to the onset of this belief, he had been
good friends with his neighbours and collateral history indicates that he has nothing
to fear from them. Besides the presence of this delusional belief, his mental state
examination is unremarkable. What is the probable diagnosis?

(a) Alzheimer's disease
(b) Paranoid schizophrenia
(c) Severe depression with psychotic symptoms
(d) Paranoid personality disorder
(e) **Delusional disorder**

This man has presented with a monothematic delusional disorder, with
a persecutory theme. There are no other psychotic symptoms evident
and no mood symptoms detected, thus excluding a diagnosis of paranoid
schizophrenia or severe depression with psychotic symptoms. The
mental state examination is otherwise unremarkable, ruling out cognitive
impairment, which is seen in Alzheimer's disease. The man has held
this delusional belief for the past year. Paranoid personality disorder is a
lifelong disorder, in which an individual might believe that others have
malign intentions towards them, but these beliefs do not reach delusional
intensity/conviction. See WHO (1992).

15 You are called to the emergency department to review a 25-year-old man. He was
brought to the emergency department by ambulance after being found unconscious
in his front garden. He had taken an overdose of codeine and benzodiazepines in
response to second-person command hallucinations and claims that he is no longer
able to resist their instructions. He has had no previous contact with psychiatric
services. He is now medically stable. What is the most appropriate management
intervention?

(a) Recommend treatment with antipsychotic medication and discharge for out-
patient follow-up over the next week
(b) Arrange for the patient to be followed up at home in the coming days by the
community mental health team
(c) Admit to the medical ward of the hospital
(d) **Admission to the psychiatric unit of the hospital**
(e) Recommend treatment with an SSRI and discharge for out-patient follow-up
over the next week

This is a first-episode-psychosis presentation in a patient with no history of
mental illness. This man has presented to the emergency department after a
suicide attempt that occurred when he acted on instructions received from
command hallucinations. The priority here is ensuring the safety of the
patient and protecting him from any immediate risk of harming himself.
This will require a hospital admission. This patient should be admitted
to hospital, under Mental Health Act legislation if required, where a

comprehensive diagnostic assessment can be completed. This will direct the appropriate treatment with either antipsychotic or antidepressant medication (or a combination of both).

Death from suicide is 12 times higher in first-episode psychosis compared with in the general population. Suicide accounts for approximately 2–5% of deaths in patients with first-episode psychosis, with the risk being greatest soon after presentation. Suicide risk is increased in those with a diagnosis of psychotic depression (which is an important differential in this case) and command hallucinations are thought to further increase that risk. See Dutta *et al* (2010) and Pompili *et al* (2011).

16 A 25-year-old man presents to the clinic with a 1-year history of functional decline and psychotic symptoms. He presents with third-person auditory hallucinations that give a running commentary on his thoughts and actions, bizarre delusions, including believing that he is the father of the Queen of England, and describes thought withdrawal. He displays formal thought disorder, with derailment and neologisms prominent. He has experienced recurrent episodes of mood disturbance for extended periods over the past 2 years and currently displays features of mania. He intermittently uses cannabis and previously used amphetamines, but stopped 6 months ago. What is the probable diagnosis?

(a) Paranoid schizophrenia
(b) Drug-induced psychosis
(c) Delusional disorder
(d) **Schizoaffective disorder**
(e) Bipolar affective disorder

Schizoaffective disorder is diagnosed when the patient has features of both schizophrenia and a mood disorder but does not strictly meet the diagnostic criteria for either illness alone. In this case, the patient is presenting with Schneiderian first-rank symptoms but also mood symptoms, which have occurred concurrent to the psychotic symptoms. In ICD-10, schizoaffective disorder is diagnosed by simultaneous and equally prominent mood and psychotic symptoms, particularly the occurrence of Schneiderian first-rank symptoms in the context of prominent mood disturbance. The term should not be applied to patients who exhibit schizophrenic symptoms and mood symptoms only in different episodes of illness. See WHO (1992).

17 A 26-year-old woman has been diagnosed with a first episode of paranoid schizophrenia. Which of the following is the most appropriate treatment option?
(a) Flupentixol decanoate
(b) **Olanzapine**
(c) Fluoxetine
(d) Diazepam
(e) Lithium carbonate

Oral antipsychotic medication is the first-line pharmacotherapeutic option in this case. Generally, second-generation atypical antipsychotics are first prescribed.

Flupentixol decanoate is a depot medication and would not be used as a first-line treatment option in paranoid schizophrenia nor would it be recommended for use in an individual who is antipsychotic naive, because of increased risks of adverse events, particularly extrapyramidal side-effects. Fluoxetine is an SSRI antidepressant, lithium carbonate is a mood stabiliser indicated for use in affective disorders, and diazepam is a benzodiazepine, which is an anxiolytic agent; none of these would be indicated as a first-line treatment for paranoid schizophrenia. See Taylor *et al* (2012).

18 A 27-year-old man was reviewed at the clinic by the consultant psychiatrist with you in attendance. The consultant psychiatrist informed you that the patient had a diagnosis of treatment-resistant schizophrenia. What is a recognised diagnostic criterion for treatment-resistant schizophrenia?

(a)   No antipsychotic medication is effective
(b)   Only injectable antipsychotic medication is effective
(c)   Lack of clinical response to trials of two different low-dose antipsychotics
(d)   **Lack of clinical response to two different antipsychotics at optimal dose and for sufficient duration**
(e)   Lack of clinical response to antipsychotic medication because of comorbid affective disorder

Treatment-resistant schizophrenia is defined as follows: An insufficient response to two clinical trials of 4 or 6 weeks' duration using monotherapy with two different antipsychotics, at least one of which should be a second generation if available. Treatment-resistant schizophrenia is estimated to affect 30% of those with schizophrenia. Clozapine is the only efficacious and licensed antipsychotic treatment for treatment-resistant schizophrenia. However, clozapine treatment will still only improve symptoms in 40–70% of these patients. See Taylor *et al* (2012).

19 A 26-year-old man attends the clinic with a history of unremitting psychotic symptoms since the onset of his illness 1 year ago. He has been treated with three different antipsychotics, olanzapine (20 mg daily), risperidone (6 mg daily) and haloperidol (15 mg daily), without achieving a therapeutic response. The consultant on the team asks you to review the patient's presentation and history to exclude comorbid features that might be leading to the treatment resistance/non-response. All the following can impact on antipsychotic treatment response, except:

(a)   **Marital status**
(b)   Comorbid depression
(c)   Alcohol misuse
(d)   Medication non-adherence
(e)   Recurring stressor

Antipsychotic treatment resistance can only be identified when a patient has been treated with an optimal/therapeutic dose of antipsychotic medication. It is also important to recognise that a therapeutic antipsychotic dose might not be tolerated by a patient because of the occurrence of side-effects, which might in turn lead to treatment non-adherence and the appearance of treatment non-response. It is important to recognise treatment resistance early, in order that inappropriate use of other antipsychotic medications instead of clozapine is avoided and that clozapine treatment can be started without unnecessary delay. See Taylor *et al* (2012).

20 A 25-year-old woman attends the early intervention service for the treatment of first-episode psychosis. All the following are recommended interventions in first-episode psychosis, except:

    (a)   Cognitive–behavioural therapy
    (b)   Family involvement and support
    (c)   **High-dose antipsychotic medication**
    (d)   Educational and vocational rehabilitation
    (e)   Relapse prevention strategy

First-episode psychosis is a heterogeneous group of diagnoses that is not synonymous with a diagnosis of schizophrenia. Typically, within a group of these patients, around 25% have bipolar disorder or psychotic depression, and only 30–40% will meet criteria for schizophrenia at presentation, although this proportion will increase over time. Approximately 50–60% of individuals with first-episode psychosis will eventually be diagnosed with schizophrenia, but others present with acute and transient psychotic disorders, substance-induced psychosis and psychotic mood disorders. Low-dose antipsychotic medication is a recommended first-line pharmacotherapeutic intervention.

Robust psychosocial interventions, delivered in an assertive outreach model of care, in conjunction with antipsychotic medication, have been shown to be effective in first-episode psychosis. Cognitive–behavioural therapy, vocational rehabilitation, a consistent key worker for the patient, family support, support with reducing/controlling substance and alcohol use, and supporting the patient in developing relapse prevention strategies are all key components of an effective early intervention service for first-episode psychosis. It is worth noting that the evidence base for the effectiveness of cognitive–behavioural therapy in schizophrenia is limited, with meta-analyses indicating that only small effects on overall symptoms are found and that non-significant effects are found on positive symptoms when trials are blinded. See Jauhar *et al* (2014) and Spencer *et al* (2001).

EMI answers

Diagnosis

Options:

(a) Paranoid schizophrenia
(b) Delusional disorder, somatic type
(c) Manic episode with mood-congruent psychotic features
(d) Delusional misidentification
(e) Schizoaffective disorder
(f) Substance-induced psychotic disorder
(g) Delusional disorder, persecutory type
(h) Severe depressive episode with mood-congruent psychotic features

For each of the following clinical vignettes, please select the probable diagnosis.

1 A 25-year-old man complains that he is being spied on by the intelligence services. He reports that his house is bugged and that he can hear agents speaking about what he is doing. He is convinced that this is happening and states that it started 6 months ago.

(a) Paranoid schizophrenia

2 A 64-year-old woman presents to her GP with multiple physical complaints. She reports that she has felt tired and exhausted for the past few months. She tells her GP that her 'body is dead' and that she can hear her dead husband calling her to join him.

(h) Severe depressive episode with mood-congruent psychotic features

3 A 22-year-old woman presents to the emergency department, reporting that her college classmates wish to kill her. She is highly distressed and agitated. She became acutely aware of this threat to her safety 2 days previously and reports that, since then, she has been hiding in her bedroom with a knife to protect herself. She reports that she has heard the voices of her classmates discussing her and laughing about her. She had used amphetamines 4 days ago.

(f) Substance-induced psychotic disorder

Treatment choices

Options:

(a) Stop clozapine
(b) Start hyoscine hydrobromide
(c) Reduce clozapine
(d) Add antidepressant
(e) Start depot medication
(f) Increase clozapine
(g) Admit to hospital
(h) Add amisulpride

Select an intervention that would be recommended for each of the following clinical scenarios.

1 A 33-year-old woman, treated with clozapine in the community, presents reporting reduced energy over the past month. She reports feeling low, has lost interest in day-to-day activities, is sleeping poorly and reports poor concentration.

(d) Add antidepressant

2 A 28-year-old man is being titrated with clozapine. He complains that his pillow is soaking wet when he wakes in the morning.

(b) Start hyoscine hydrobromide

3 A 30-year-old man has been treated with clozapine for 6 months. He reports that he stopped smoking cigarettes 2 weeks ago. Today he seems sedated and reports that he has been constipated over the past week.

(c) Reduce clozapine

Treatment choices

Options:

(a) Quetiapine
(b) Depot medication
(c) Electroconvulsive therapy
(d) Lamotrigine
(e) Clozapine
(f) Antidepressant medication
(g) Hospital admission
(h) Lithium carbonate

Select an intervention that would be recommended for each of the following clinical scenarios.

1 A 26-year-old woman with a diagnosis of schizophrenia is admitted to hospital following a relapse of psychosis. This is her third hospitalisation in the past year and all have occurred secondary to non-adherence to oral antipsychotic medication. She had previously responded to oral antipsychotic medication when adherent.

(b) Depot medication

2 A 34-year-old man with a diagnosis of schizophrenia presents to A&E reporting command hallucinations and suicidal thoughts.

(g) Hospital admission

3 A 28-year-old man with a history of schizophrenia presents to the clinic with ongoing psychotic symptoms, having failed to respond to three different antipsychotic treatments.

(e) Clozapine

CHAPTER 3

Depression and anxiety disorders

MCQs

1 You have been treating a 40-year-old man with a first episode of a depressive illness over the past 8 weeks. He is currently on sertraline 100 mg once daily, has responded well to the treatment and is currently asymptomatic. What is the most appropriate way to proceed with his management?

   (a) Reduce and gradually discontinue his antidepressant
   (b) Reduce to a lower dose of 50 mg once daily
   (c) Increase the dose to 150 mg once daily
   (d) Continue with 100 mg once daily for 3 months, then discontinue
   (e) Continue with 100 mg once daily for 6 months, then discontinue

2 With regard to the epidemiology of depression, which one of the following statements is correct?

   (a) Equally common in males and females
   (b) The mean age at onset is in the mid-40s
   (c) Suicide rate of 40%
   (d) Lower prevalence than bipolar affective disorder
   (e) Lifetime risk of 15%

3 A 35-year-old married man is referred to the emergency department for an assessment of his depressive illness. Which of the following would indicate that a hospital admission would be required?

   (a) Insomnia
   (b) Anhedonia
   (c) Worthlessness
   (d) Distressing auditory hallucinations
   (e) Poor concentration

4   A 25-year-old woman is referred to the out-patient clinic by her GP. She describes the following symptoms: pervasively low mood and anxiety for the past month, low energy, poor concentration and insomnia. No other depressive symptoms are elicited. She has no history of depressive episodes and is requesting that a treatment intervention be offered. Which of the following would be the most appropriate first-line treatment?

    (a)   Zopiclone
    (b)   Mirtazapine
    (c)   Diazepam
    (d)   Cognitive–behavioural therapy
    (e)   Psychodynamic psychotherapy

5   A 56-year-old man is seen at the out-patient clinic. He presents with low mood following the death of his wife 2 months previously. All the following features are more consistent with a depressive episode than with a normal bereavement reaction, except:

    (a)   Psychomotor retardation
    (b)   Suicidal ideation
    (c)   Insomnia
    (d)   Delusions of poverty
    (e)   Impaired social and occupational functioning

6   A 25-year-old woman with a diagnosis of OCD is attending the clinic. She has been treated with fluoxetine 20 mg daily for the past 3 months but with no improvement in her symptoms. Which of these is the most appropriate next step?

    (a)   Switch to a different SSRI
    (b)   Increase the dose of fluoxetine
    (c)   Add an atypical antipsychotic
    (d)   Add clonazepam
    (e)   Switch to venlafaxine

7   A 22-year-old man presents to his GP in a highly distressed state. He reports experiencing recurrent intrusive thoughts and images of him hitting someone. Such an aggressive act, he says, would be completely out of character for him. He acknowledges that the thoughts and images are 'stupid' and senseless, but is unable to completely stop them from entering his mind. He recognises the thoughts as his own. He describes heightened anxiety associated with the thoughts and images. What is the probable diagnosis?

    (a)   OCD with prominent obsessional symptoms
    (b)   Dissocial personality disorder with poor impulse control
    (c)   No mental illness
    (d)   Avoidant/anxious personality disorder
    (e)   Generalised anxiety disorder

8   A 22-year-old college student presents to the clinic reporting worry regarding an exam that she must take in a week. She has had low energy, poor concentration, insomnia and 'always feels under pressure' for over 2 years. She recently saw a neurologist because she was worried that her frequent headaches and muscle tension meant that she had a neurological illness. The neurologist assured her that she didn't have a neurological illness, which reassured her. What is the most probable diagnosis?

(a)   Generalised anxiety disorder
(b)   Hypochondriasis
(c)   Depression
(d)   Somatisation disorder
(e)   Adjustment disorder

9   A 21-year-old woman is attending the clinic for the first time. She is currently repeating her university examinations for the third consecutive year. She reports being unable to attend lectures and seminars because she feels 'anxious' while attending them. She dreads being asked a question in front of the group as she is concerned that she will say something stupid. She has been unable to make friends as she avoids conversation out of fear that she will have to talk to more than one person. She constantly worries about others judging her when in conversation and as a result avoids mixing with people as much as she can. She finds relief from her anxiety symptoms when at home. What is the probable diagnosis?

(a)   Generalised anxiety disorder
(b)   Social phobia
(c)   Paranoid personality disorder
(d)   No mental disorder
(e)   Delusional disorder

10 A 25-year-old woman with a diagnosis of panic disorder is attending the clinic for her first psychotherapy session. You plan to provide psychoeducation to her about the nature of panic attacks. Which of the following is not true about panic attacks:

(a)   Panic attacks involve a misinterpretation of bodily symptoms
(b)   Panic attacks generally last for up to 1 h
(c)   Panic attacks are generally harmless to your physical health
(d)   Panic attacks do not usually occur in response to real danger
(e)   Panic attacks usually do not involve fainting episodes

11 A 20-year-old college student attends the emergency department, reporting palpitations and chest tightness. He is highly distressed, urging nursing staff to do something to help him and telling them he's having a heart attack. This is the third episode of this kind he has had in the past week, and he has had more over the previous 6 months. He also experiences a sensation of choking during these episodes; he hyperventilates and feels as if he will pass out. He is reviewed by an emergency department doctor, who fails to identify any evidence on electrocardiogram or in laboratory studies to indicate that the patient had experienced a myocardial infarction or other cardiac event. You assess the patient and diagnose him with panic disorder. All the following concerning panic disorder are true: except

(a) Depression does not commonly occur with panic disorder
(b) Lifetime prevalence rates of alcohol and substance misuse disorders are increased in panic disorder
(c) Patients with panic disorder who have a concurrent depression have a higher risk of suicide attempts
(d) Panic disorder can often be associated with a fear of travelling on your own
(e) Individuals with panic disorder are more likely to seek medical assistance than individuals with other anxiety disorders

12 A 45-year-old man is attending the clinic and wishes to discuss his diagnosis of recurrent depressive disorder. He has recently returned to work on a part-time basis. He is concerned that, if he were to experience a further episode of depression, he might have to leave his job. Which is the most significant risk factor for relapse in a patient with recurrent depressive disorder?

(a) Older age of the patient
(b) The dose of antidepressant needed for response
(c) Gender of the patient
(d) Family history of depression
(e) Residual symptoms

13 A 32-year-old mother of one attends the clinic 2 months postpartum. She presents with low mood for the past 6 weeks, marked anxiety, guilty ideation, insomnia, early-morning wakening, loss of appetite, anhedonia and low energy. She worries that she is an incapable mother and has become more reliant on her own mother to help with childcare. She denies suicidal or homicidal ideation. What is the most likely diagnosis?

(a) Mild depressive episode
(b) Moderate depressive episode with onset in the postpartum period
(c) Baby blues
(d) Normal adjustment reaction
(e) Postpartum psychosis

14 A 70-year-old woman is admitted to hospital for treatment of psychotic depression. The clinical record made at the time of her admission describes her presentation as: 'She presents with a severely depressed mood, with marked negative cognitions and mood-congruent delusions.' Which of the following would not be consistent with the description of a mood-congruent delusion in this case?

(a) Delusions of poverty
(b) Delusions of guilt
(c) Delusions of thought broadcasting
(d) Hypochondriacal delusions
(e) Nihilistic delusions

15 A 35-year-old woman attends the clinic reporting increased stress and anxiety, having been involved in a road traffic accident some 3 months previously. She wishes to know if she has PTSD. Which of the following symptoms are not indicative of PTSD?

(a) Nightmares
(b) Avoidance of travelling in cars
(c) Physiological arousal on reminders of the accident
(d) Hypervigilance
(e) Persecutory delusions

16 A 35-year-old retired soldier is referred to your clinic for assessment and treatment of PTSD. Which of the following is not a recommended treatment for PTSD?

(a) Cognitive–behavioural therapy
(b) Fluoxetine
(c) Eye movement desensitisation and reprocessing
(d) Diazepam
(e) Sertraline

17 A 40-year-old man has been assessed at the clinic and diagnosed with a moderate depressive episode. He has expressed a preference for antidepressant therapy. All the following should be considered in making a medication choice, except:

(a) Prescribing an antidepressant with a rapid onset of action
(b) The patient's prior experience with antidepressant medication
(c) Toxicity of antidepressant in overdose for patients at risk of suicide
(d) Concurrent medical conditions
(e) Concurrent medication use

18 A 35-year-old woman has returned to the clinic today having been treated with sertraline 100 mg daily for a moderate depressive episode for the past 8 weeks. Her depressive episode began 6 months ago. Her depressive symptoms have worsened since her last appointment. She has refused psychological therapy. Which of the following would not be considered an appropriate management strategy at this time?

(a) Switching to another antidepressant from a different pharmacological class
(b) Combining two antidepressants from different classes
(c) Combining the antidepressant with a psychotherapeutic intervention
(d) Discontinuing all antidepressant therapy because of its lack of efficacy
(e) Augmenting the antidepressant with other agents to increase its efficacy

19 While observing a patient consultation, a senior clinician remarks that the patient just assessed had marked features of the somatic syndrome (i.e. biological symptoms of depression) associated with depression. Which of the following is found in the somatic syndrome in depression, as defined by the ICD-10 diagnostic criteria?

(a) Poor concentration
(b) Diurnal mood variation
(c) Low self-esteem
(d) Suicidal ideation
(e) Constipation

20 A 28-year-old woman is attending the clinic 2 months after giving birth to her first child. She has a diagnosis of postpartum depression. From the history you establish the patient had a number of risk factors for postpartum depression. Which of the following is not a risk factor for the development of postpartum depression?

(a) Past history of depression
(b) Depression during the pregnancy
(c) Being married
(d) Recent stressful life events
(e) Anxiety disorder during the pregnancy

EMI questions

Diagnosis

Options:

    (a) Generalised anxiety disorder
    (b) OCD
    (c) Social phobia
    (d) Depressive episode
    (e) Delusional disorder
    (f) Panic disorder
    (g) Agoraphobia
    (h) PTSD

For each of the following clinical vignettes, please select the probable diagnosis.

1   A 22-year-old college student attends the clinic, reporting unbearable embarrassment and tension when asked to speak in groups. She has stopped attending classes because of fears that she will be asked to answer a question in front of the class. She believes that she is been judged by peers when socialising and avoids mixing with her classmates as a result.

2   A 30-year-old man presents at the clinic, reporting 'not having enough time in the day'. He rarely leaves his house because of the long periods of time that he spends cleaning his kitchen and bathroom. He has constant thoughts and fears about becoming infected by germs and finds these thoughts to be anxiety-inducing.

3   A 30-year-old woman presents to the clinic reporting that she feels exhausted. She describes poor concentration and sleep and that she feels on edge most of time, making it difficult for her to switch off. She reports experiencing muscle tension and recurrent headaches. This has been occurring for nearly a year now and she is frustrated by feeling unable to cope with daily activities and being worried about most things on a daily basis.

Treatment options

Options:

    (a) Fluoxetine
    (b) Psychodynamic psychotherapy
    (c) Cognitive–behavioural therapy
    (d) Olanzapine
    (e) Amitriptyline
    (f) Electroconvulsive therapy
    (g) Exposure and response prevention therapy
    (h) Diazepam

Select an intervention that would be recommended for each of the following clinical scenarios. (There may be more than one answer for some of the questions.)

1   A 30-year-old woman has a 3-month history of a loss of interest in day-to-day activities and a loss of enjoyment in family interaction. She reports that she is waking 2 h earlier than normal in the mornings and that she feels worse at that time of the day. She finds it difficult to sustain her attention and has noticed herself being more forgetful. She has tended to blame herself for trivial mistakes over this time. (Select two options.)

2   A 42-year-old man has been referred to the clinic by his GP. He reports a long-standing sense of failure and that he is never satisfied with life. He says that he was never appreciated by his father and that he would like to get to the bottom of this. (Select one option.)

3   You attend a patient's house with a community mental health nurse to review a patient who is struggling to leave the house to attend appointments. He spends long periods of time checking that all electrical appliances are switched off and that the doors and windows are locked before being able to consider leaving home. This often involves him spending hours every day performing these checks. Eventually, he resigns himself to staying in, as that helps him to feel less anxious. (Select two options.)

Diagnosis

Options:
- (a)   Depression
- (b)   Panic disorder
- (c)   Generalised anxiety disorder
- (d)   Agoraphobia
- (e)   OCD
- (f)   Adjustment disorder
- (g)   Hypochondriacal disorder
- (h)   PTSD

For each of the following clinical vignettes, please select the probable diagnosis.

1   A 30-year-old woman returns to her GP, reporting that she is certain that she has skin cancer. She requests further investigations in order to confirm the diagnosis. This is despite her GP having performed the appropriate tests previously and referred her to a dermatologist for a second opinion. The GP continues to reassure her that she doesn't have cancer. Despite the reassurance she remains anxious that she has skin cancer and continues to attend the GP surgery requesting further investigations.

2   A 25-year-old woman presents to the clinic with a 3-month history of angry outbursts and feeling fearful and on edge all the time. She was involved in a road traffic accident 6 months ago and finds herself reliving the accident over and over again.

3   A 45-year-old woman is accompanied to the clinic by her sister. She has not left her house alone for the past 9 months. She describes heightened anxiety when leaving the house alone and had experienced two episodes of panic while in a local shop a year ago. She describes being afraid of not being able to find an exit when in public. She denies having had any further episodes of panic since that time.

MCQ answers

1   You have been treating a 40-year-old man with a first episode of a depressive illness over the past 8 weeks. He is currently on sertraline 100 mg once daily, has responded well to the treatment and is currently asymptomatic. What is the most appropriate way to proceed with his management?
   (a)   Reduce and gradually discontinue his antidepressant
   (b)   Reduce to a lower dose of 50 mg once daily
   (c)   Increase the dose to 150 mg once daily
   (d)   Continue with 100 mg once daily for 3 months, then discontinue
   (e)   **Continue with 100 mg once daily for 6 months, then discontinue**

An individual's response to antidepressant therapy is heterogenous in terms of long-term remission. After commencing antidepressant treatment, there is usually a delay of 7–10 days before a discernible response emerges. Evidence of an antidepressant effect is most likely to occur within the first 2 weeks of treatment. The recommendation is for continued antidepressant treatment for 6–9 months subsequent to a full response being gained (i.e. subsequent to patient becoming asymptomatic). See Malhi *et al* (2013) and Taylor *et al* (2012).

2   With regard to the epidemiology of depression, which one of the following statements is correct?
   (a)   Equally common in males and females
   (b)   The mean age at onset is in the mid-40s
   (c)   Suicide rate of 40%
   (d)   Lower prevalence than bipolar affective disorder
   (e)   **Lifetime risk of 15%**

About 15% of people will have a depressive episode at some point during their lifetime. The average age at onset of depression (25–35 years) is approximately 10 years older than for bipolar affective disorder. Females have an approximately twofold increase in depression risk compared with males. See Frank & Thase (1999).

3   A 35-year-old married man is referred to the emergency department for an assessment of his depressive illness. Which of the following would indicate that a hospital admission would be required?

   (a)   Insomnia
   (b)   Anhedonia
   (c)   Worthlessness
   (d)   **Distressing auditory hallucinations**
   (e)   Poor concentration

The presence of auditory hallucinations would categorise this man's presentation as a severe depressive episode with psychotic symptoms. The other symptoms can occur along with hallucinations in a psychotic depression, but these symptoms in themselves do not suffice to diagnose psychotic depression. The presence of auditory hallucinations indicates that the illness has progressed to a stage where the patient's reality testing is impaired.

Patients with psychotic major depression demonstrate significantly more severe psychomotor disturbances (retardation or agitation) and increased suicidal ideation than do patients with non-psychotic depression. In-patient admission is advisable to allow for a comprehensive assessment and treatment. See WHO (1992).

4   A 25-year-old woman is referred to the out-patient clinic by her GP. She describes the following symptoms: pervasively low mood and anxiety for the past month, low energy, poor concentration and insomnia. No other depressive symptoms are elicited. She has no history of depressive episodes and is requesting that a treatment intervention be offered. Which of the following would be the most appropriate first-line treatment?

   (a)   Zopiclone
   (b)   Mirtazapine
   (c)   Diazepam
   (d)   **Cognitive–behavioural therapy**
   (e)   Psychodynamic psychotherapy

This woman is having a mild depressive episode, according to ICD-10 criteria. Four symptoms are required for a diagnosis of mild depression, six symptoms for a diagnosis of moderate depression and eight or more symptoms (or the occurrence of psychotic symptoms, specifically hallucinations, delusions or depressive stupor) for a diagnosis of a severe depressive episode.

There are a number of therapeutic options for a mild depressive episode. Antidepressant medications are not first-line, although if this was a recurrent depressive episode, then an SSRI could be considered. Given that this woman has no history of depression and is requesting that a treatment intervention be provided, then a course of cognitive–behavioural therapy would be the most appropriate intervention. See NICE (2009a) and WHO (1992).

5   A 56-year-old man is seen at the out-patient clinic. He presents with low mood
    following the death of his wife 2 months previously. All the following features are
    more consistent with a depressive episode than with a normal bereavement reaction,
    except:

    (a)   Psychomotor retardation
    (b)   Suicidal ideation
    (c)   **Insomnia**
    (d)   Delusions of poverty
    (e)   Impaired social and occupational functioning

An uncomplicated bereavement reaction ends within 2 months, is not
markedly impairing and includes no suicidal ideation, no psychomotor
retardation, and no morbid sense of worthlessness. Unlike the other
symptoms of a major depressive disorder, these last three symptoms
are uncharacteristic of normal distress and thus are likely to indicate
a depressive disorder. The presence of delusional guilt or delusions of
poverty would also indicate a severe depressive illness rather than a normal
bereavement reaction. See Wakefield & Schmitz (2013).

6   A 25-year-old woman with a diagnosis of OCD is attending the clinic. She has been
    treated with fluoxetine 20 mg daily for the past 3 months but with no improvement
    in her symptoms. Which of these is the most appropriate next step?

    (a)   Switch to a different SSRI
    (b)   **Increase the dose of fluoxetine**
    (c)   Add an atypical antipsychotic
    (d)   Add clonazepam
    (e)   Switch to venlafaxine

The two first-line treatments for OCD are pharmacotherapy and cognitive–
behavioural therapy using exposure and response prevention (ERP).
Medications that are predominantly serotonergic (i.e. acting to promote
serotonergic function), such as SSRIs, venlafaxine and some tricyclic
antidepressants (e.g. clomipramine) are the most effective. Before starting
an SSRI for the treatment of OCD, the patient should be informed that
a significant treatment response can take up to 6–8 weeks to occur (and
sometimes 10–12 weeks for a full response). Higher doses (e.g. fluoxetine
at 40 mg or 60 mg daily) are more effective in OCD.

   An SSRI alone is a reasonable initial treatment for a patient who has
responded to a given medication in a previous trial, or is unable to cooperate
with cognitive–behavioural therapy, or prefers this treatment. ERP is
indicated for a patient who prefers to avoid medications and is willing to
do the work of ERP. Combining an SSRI and ERP can be more effective
than monotherapy for some patients, such as those with moderate–severe
disease. See Fineberg & Brown (2011).

7   A 22-year-old man presents to his GP in a highly distressed state. He reports experienc-
    ing recurrent intrusive thoughts and images of him hitting someone. Such an aggressive
    act, he says, would be completely out of character for him. He acknowledges that the
    thoughts and images are 'stupid' and senseless, but is unable to completely stop them
    from entering his mind. He recognises the thoughts as his own. He describes heightened
    anxiety associated with the thoughts and images. What is the probable diagnosis?

    (a)   **OCD with prominent obsessional symptoms**
    (b)   Dissocial personality disorder with poor impulse control
    (c)   No mental illness
    (d)   Avoidant/anxious personality disorder
    (e)   Generalised anxiety disorder

This patient has features of OCD with prominent obsessions concerning
him acting aggressively. Obsessions are recurrent and persistent thoughts,
impulses, images or doubts that are experienced during the disturbance, are
experienced as intrusive and inappropriate and can cause marked anxiety
or distress. This distress distinguishes OCD from anankastic personality
disorder, where obsessional symptoms are often 'egosyntonic'. The
thoughts, impulses or images are not simply excessive worries about real-
life problems. The patient attempts to ignore or suppress such thoughts,
impulses or images, or to neutralise them with some other thought or
action. The patient recognises that they are a product of their own mind
(not imposed from outside, as in thought insertion). See Koran (2007).

8   A 22-year-old college student presents to the clinic reporting worry regarding an exam
    that she must take in a week. She has had low energy, poor concentration, insomnia
    and 'always feels under pressure' for over 2 years. She recently saw a neurologist
    because she was worried that her frequent headaches and muscle tension meant
    that she had a neurological illness. The neurologist assured her that she didn't have
    a neurological illness, which reassured her. What is the most probable diagnosis?

    (a)   **Generalised anxiety disorder**
    (b)   Hypochondriasis
    (c)   Depression
    (d)   Somatisation disorder
    (e)   Adjustment disorder

Generalised anxiety disorder is relatively common, with a lifetime prevalence
of about 5–8%. It is hallmarked by what is described as 'free-floating'
anxiety, meaning that an individual will worry about many different
things without there being a specific focus or theme to their concerns.
The patient with generalised anxiety disorder will also have a wide range
of symptoms relating to the degree of anxiety, including low energy, poor
concentration, insomnia, irritability, muscle tension and feeling unable
to relax, and will generally experience significant functional impairment.
There is a significant level of psychiatric comorbidity (e.g. high prevalence
of comorbid depression). ICD-10 diagnostic criteria require that symptoms
have persisted for 6 months or more for a diagnosis of generalised anxiety
disorder to be made. See Hoge *et al* (2012).

9   A 21-year-old woman is attending the clinic for the first time. She is currently repeating her university examinations for the third consecutive year. She reports being unable to attend lectures and seminars because she feels 'anxious' while attending them. She dreads being asked a question in front of the group as she is concerned that she will say something stupid. She has been unable to make friends as she avoids conversation out of fear that she will have to talk to more than one person. She constantly worries about others judging her when in conversation and as a result avoids mixing with people as much as she can. She finds relief from her anxiety symptoms when at home. What is the probable diagnosis?

(a)   Generalised anxiety disorder
(b)   **Social phobia**
(c)   Paranoid personality disorder
(d)   No mental disorder
(e)   Delusional disorder

Social phobia (also known as social anxiety disorder) is defined as a marked and persistent fear of social or performance situations. Individuals with social phobia fear that they will act in a way that will be embarrassing. They fear being evaluated in social situations and such situations engender high levels of anxiety for the individual. Untreated, social phobia can persist for many years and is associated with comorbid psychiatric disorders. Epidemiological studies have demonstrated a lifetime prevalence of 12%. See Vriends *et al* (2014).

10 A 25-year-old woman with a diagnosis of panic disorder is attending the clinic for her first psychotherapy session. You plan to provide psychoeducation to her about the nature of panic attacks. Which of the following is not true about panic attacks:

(a)   Panic attacks involve a misinterpretation of bodily symptoms
(b)   **Panic attacks generally last for up to 1 h**
(c)   Panic attacks are generally harmless to your physical health
(d)   Panic attacks do not usually occur in response to real danger
(e)   Panic attacks usually do not involve fainting episodes

Panic attacks represent the body's 'fight–flight–freeze' response kicking in. This response prepares our body to defend itself (e.g. our heart beats faster to pump blood to our muscles, so that we have the energy to run away or fight off danger). However, sometimes our body reacts when there is no real danger. The patient experiencing panic attacks will misinterpret bodily sensations associated with the fight–flight–freeze response as dangerous; for example, believing that an increase in your heart rate means that you are having a heart attack. Panic attacks are brief (typically lasting only 5–10 min at peak intensity) and, although extremely uncomfortable and frightening, are harmless to a person physically. See Royal College of Psychiatrists (2013).

11 A 20-year-old college student attends the emergency department, reporting palpitations and chest tightness. He is highly distressed, urging nursing staff to do something to help him and telling them he's having a heart attack. This is the third episode of this kind he has had in the past week, and he has had more over the previous 6 months. He also experiences a sensation of choking during these episodes; he hyperventilates and feels as if he will pass out. He is reviewed by an emergency department doctor, who fails to identify any evidence on electrocardiogram or in laboratory studies to indicate that the patient had experienced a myocardial infarction or other cardiac event. You assess the patient and diagnose him with panic disorder. All the following concerning panic disorder are true: except

(a) **Depression does not commonly occur with panic disorder**
(b) Lifetime prevalence rates of alcohol and substance misuse disorders are increased in panic disorder
(c) Patients with panic disorder who have a concurrent depression have a higher risk of suicide attempts
(d) Panic disorder can often be associated with a fear of travelling on your own
(e) Individuals with panic disorder are more likely to seek medical assistance than individuals with other anxiety disorders

The lifetime prevalence of panic disorder is approximately 2%, and is approximately twice as high in women as in men. The lifetime prevalence of depression as a comorbid diagnosis with panic disorder is approximately 50–60%. Panic disorder is associated with agoraphobia in approximately 20% of cases. Given the increased risk of suicidal ideation and suicide completion with depression, the risk of suicide in panic disorder is higher with comorbid depression. See Barr Taylor (2006).

12 A 45-year-old man is attending the clinic and wishes to discuss his diagnosis of recurrent depressive disorder. He has recently returned to work on a part-time basis. He is concerned that, if he were to experience a further episode of depression, he might have to leave his job. Which is the most significant risk factor for relapse in a patient with recurrent depressive disorder?

(a) Older age of the patient
(b) The dose of antidepressant needed for response
(c) Gender of the patient
(d) Family history of depression
(e) **Residual symptoms**

There are a number of risk factors associated with the risk of relapse in recurrent depressive disorder, including residual depressive symptoms (i.e. persisting sub-syndromal or syndromal depressive symptoms, meaning that the patient has not had a complete response to treatment), younger age at onset, psychotic symptoms, the severity of depressive symptoms, and the number of prior depressive episodes. See Burcusa & Iacono (2007).

13 A 32-year-old mother of one attends the clinic 2 months postpartum. She presents with low mood for the past 6 weeks, marked anxiety, guilty ideation, insomnia, early-morning wakening, loss of appetite, anhedonia and low energy. She worries that she is an incapable mother and has become more reliant on her own mother to help with childcare. She denies suicidal or homicidal ideation. What is the most likely diagnosis?

  (a) Mild depressive episode
  (b) **Moderate depressive episode with onset in the postpartum period**
  (c) Baby blues
  (d) Normal adjustment reaction
  (e) Postpartum psychosis

Postpartum depression presents with depressed mood, irritability, anhedonia, insomnia, fatigue, anxiety, guilt, concerns about an inability to care for the child, thoughts of suicide, and in severe cases it can lead to maternal suicide and infanticide. It affects approximately 10–15% of women in the first year following delivery. In this case the patient is presenting with six symptoms of a depressive illness, indicating that she is experiencing a moderate depressive episode with onset within the postpartum period (i.e. within 1 month of giving birth).

Postpartum or baby blues are the most common observed puerperal mood disturbance, with estimates of prevalence ranging from 30–75%. The symptoms begin within a few days of delivery, usually on day 3 or 4, and persist for hours up to several days. The symptoms include mood lability, irritability, tearfulness, anxiety, and sleep disturbance. Postpartum blues are by definition time-limited and mild and do not require treatment other than reassurance. Severe postpartum blues are a risk factor for the later emergence of postpartum depression. See Musters *et al* (2008) and NICE (2009*b*).

14 A 70-year-old woman is admitted to hospital for treatment of psychotic depression. The clinical record made at the time of her admission describes her presentation as: 'She presents with a severely depressed mood, with marked negative cognitions and mood-congruent delusions.' Which of the following would not be consistent with the description of a mood-congruent delusion in this case?

  (a) Delusions of poverty
  (b) Delusions of guilt
  (c) **Delusions of thought broadcasting**
  (d) Hypochondriacal delusions
  (e) Nihilistic delusions

Mood-congruent delusions are identified when the content of the delusional beliefs are consistent with the pervasive mood state (depressed mood in this case) and/or underlying morbid worthlessness, overly self-deprecatory, or guilty beliefs. Mood-congruent delusions can also occur in mania, where the themes will reflect the expansiveness of the individual's mood, with grandiose delusional themes predominating. See Oyebode (2008).

15 A 35-year-old woman attends the clinic reporting increased stress and anxiety, having been involved in a road traffic accident some 3 months previously. She wishes to know if she has PTSD. Which of the following symptoms are not indicative of PTSD?

    (a)   Nightmares
    (b)   Avoidance of travelling in cars
    (c)   Physiological arousal on reminders of the accident
    (d)   Hypervigilance
    (e)   **Persecutory delusions**

PTSD is a trauma- and stress-related disorder occurring in an individual with a history of exposure to severe trauma (actual or threatened death, serious injury, or threats to the physical integrity of the self or others). In DSM-5, there are four symptom clusters described that can occur in PTSD:

▶ intrusion symptoms (formerly called re-experiencing most commonly intrusive recollections, flashbacks or dreams)

▶ alterations in arousal and reactivity (formerly called hyperarousal, and including disturbed sleep, hypervigilance and an exaggerated startle response)

▶ avoidance (e.g. efforts to avoid activities or thoughts associated with the trauma)

▶ negative alterations in cognitions and mood (e.g. emotional numbing).

PTSD is not a psychotic disorder and delusions do not occur as part of a primary PTSD diagnosis. See Ahmed (2007) and O'Donnell *et al* (2014).

16 A 35-year-old retired soldier is referred to your clinic for assessment and treatment of PTSD. Which of the following is not a recommended treatment for PTSD?

    (a)   Cognitive–behavioural therapy
    (b)   Fluoxetine
    (c)   Eye movement desensitisation and reprocessing
    (d)   **Diazepam**
    (e)   Sertraline

Psychological approaches with proven efficacy include individual trauma-focused cognitive–behavioural therapy and eye movement desensitisation and reprocessing. Trauma-focused cognitive–behavioural therapy is the recommended first-line intervention for PTSD. SSRIs, including sertraline, fluoxetine and paroxetine, are all efficacious as acute and maintenance treatment. Benzodiazepines are not recommended for the treatment of PTSD. See Ahmed (2007) and Green (2013).

17 A 40-year-old man has been assessed at the clinic and diagnosed with a moderate depressive episode. He has expressed a preference for antidepressant therapy. All the following should be considered in making a medication choice, except:

(a) **Prescribing an antidepressant with a rapid onset of action**
(b) The patient's prior experience with antidepressant medication
(c) Toxicity of antidepressant in overdose for patients at risk of suicide
(d) Concurrent medical conditions
(e) Concurrent medication use

Factors to take into account when choosing an antidepressant are the patient's prior experience with medication (including response, tolerability, adverse effects), concurrent medical conditions and use of non-psychiatric medications, possible short- and long-term side-effects, toxicity of overdose in patients at risk of suicide, the clinician's own experience with the medication, the patient's history of adherence to medication, history of first-degree relatives responding to a medication, and patient preferences. No class of antidepressant has proven to have a more rapid onset than any other. See Bauer *et al* (2013).

18 A 35-year-old woman has returned to the clinic today having been treated with sertraline 100 mg daily for a moderate depressive episode for the past 8 weeks. Her depressive episode began 6 months ago. Her depressive symptoms have worsened since her last appointment. She has refused psychological therapy. Which of the following would not be considered an appropriate management strategy at this time?

(a) Switching to another antidepressant from a different pharmacological class
(b) Combining two antidepressants from different classes
(c) Combining the antidepressant with a psychotherapeutic intervention
(d) **Discontinuing all antidepressant therapy because of its lack of efficacy**
(e) Augmenting the antidepressant with other agents to increase its efficacy

In at least 30% of depressive episodes, patients will not respond sufficiently to an adequately performed first-line treatment with any chosen antidepressant. This situation warrants a careful review of the accuracy of the diagnosis, the adequacy of antidepressant dosing, the patient's tolerability of the antidepressant, and adherence. Comorbid conditions should be assessed for and treated. An assessment for alcohol/substance misuse should be carried out.

Following this, theoretical strategies are:

▶ increasing (maximising) the dose of the initial antidepressant
▶ switching to another antidepressant in the same pharmacological class
▶ switching to another antidepressant from a different pharmacological class
▶ combining the antidepressant with a psychotherapeutic intervention
▶ combining two antidepressants from different classes
▶ augmenting the antidepressant with other agents (e.g. lithium, thyroid hormone or atypical antipsychotics) to enhance antidepressant efficacy.

See Bauer *et al* (2013).

19 While observing a patient consultation, a senior clinician remarks that the patient just assessed had marked features of the somatic syndrome (i.e. biological symptoms of depression) associated with depression. Which of the following is found in the somatic syndrome in depression, as defined by the ICD-10 diagnostic criteria?

    (a)   Poor concentration
    (b)   **Diurnal mood variation**
    (c)   Low self-esteem
    (d)   Suicidal ideation
    (e)   Constipation

Depression with somatic syndrome is synonymous with melancholic or endogenous depression. The ICD-10 diagnostic criteria require that at least four of the following are present: marked loss of interest or pleasure; loss of emotional reactivity; waking in the morning 2 h or more before usual time; depression worse in the morning (diurnal mood variation); objective evidence of marked psychomotor retardation or agitation; marked loss of appetite; weight loss (5% or more of body weight in the past month); loss of libido. See WHO (1992).

20 A 28-year-old woman is attending the clinic 2 months after giving birth to her first child. She has a diagnosis of postpartum depression. From the history you establish the patient had a number of risk factors for postpartum depression. Which of the following is not a risk factor for the development of postpartum depression?

    (a)   Past history of depression
    (b)   Depression during the pregnancy
    (c)   **Being married**
    (d)   Recent stressful life events
    (e)   Anxiety disorder during the pregnancy

Postpartum depression is defined in ICD-10 as a depressive episode that occurs within the puerperal period and defines this as within 6 weeks of the birth; DSM-5 specifies onset in the first 4 weeks after delivery. However, both these 'time of onset' criteria might be too narrow for postpartum depressive episodes. Many clinicians prefer to extend the definition to include any significant depressive episode occurring within the first year after childbirth.

Studies have consistently shown that depression or anxiety during pregnancy, recent stressful life events, poor social support and a previous history of depression are risk factors for postpartum depression. See Robertson *et al* (2004).

EMI answers

Diagnosis

Options:

(a) Generalised anxiety disorder
(b) OCD
(c) Social phobia
(d) Depressive episode
(e) Delusional disorder
(f) Panic disorder
(g) Agoraphobia
(h) PTSD

For each of the following clinical vignettes, please select the probable diagnosis.

1   A 22-year-old college student attends the clinic, reporting unbearable embarrassment and tension when asked to speak in groups. She has stopped attending classes because of fears that she will be asked to answer a question in front of the class. She believes that she is been judged by peers when socialising and avoids mixing with her classmates as a result.

(c) Social phobia

2   A 30-year-old man presents at the clinic, reporting 'not having enough time in the day'. He rarely leaves his house because of the long periods of time that he spends cleaning his kitchen and bathroom. He has constant thoughts and fears about becoming infected by germs and finds these thoughts to be anxiety-inducing.

(b) OCD

3   A 30-year-old woman presents to the clinic reporting that she feels exhausted. She describes poor concentration and sleep and that she feels on edge most of time, making it difficult for her to switch off. She reports experiencing muscle tension and recurrent headaches. This has been occurring for nearly a year now and she is frustrated by feeling unable to cope with daily activities and being worried about most things on a daily basis.

(a) Generalised anxiety disorder

Treatment options

Options:

(a) Fluoxetine
(b) Psychodynamic psychotherapy
(c) Cognitive–behavioural therapy
(d) Olanzapine
(e) Amitriptyline
(f) Electroconvulsive therapy
(g) Exposure and response prevention therapy
(h) Diazepam

Select an intervention that would be recommended for each of the following clinical scenarios. (There may be more than one answer for some of the questions.)

1 A 30-year-old woman has a 3-month history of a loss of interest in day-to-day activities and a loss of enjoyment in family interaction. She reports that she is waking 2 h earlier than normal in the mornings and that she feels worse at that time of the day. She finds it difficult to sustain her attention and has noticed herself being more forgetful. She has tended to blame herself for trivial mistakes over this time. (Select two options.)

(a) Fluoxetine

(c) Cognitive–behavioural therapy

2 A 42-year-old man has been referred to the clinic by his GP. He reports a long-standing sense of failure and that he is never satisfied with life. He says that he was never appreciated by his father and that he would like to get to the bottom of this.

(b) Psychodynamic psychotherapy

3 You attend a patient's house with a community mental health nurse to review a patient who is struggling to leave the house to attend appointments. He spends long periods of time checking that all electrical appliances are switched off and that the doors and windows are locked before being able to consider leaving home. This often involves him spending hours every day performing these checks. Eventually, he resigns himself to staying in, as that helps him to feel less anxious. (Select two options.)

(a) Fluoxetine

(g) Exposure and response prevention therapy

Diagnosis

Options:

(a) Depression
(b) Panic disorder
(c) Generalised anxiety disorder
(d) Agoraphobia
(e) OCD
(f) Adjustment disorder
(g) Hypochondriacal disorder
(h) PTSD

For each of the following clinical vignettes, please select the probable diagnosis:

1 A 30-year-old woman returns to her GP, reporting that she is certain that she has skin cancer. She requests further investigations in order to confirm the diagnosis. This is despite her GP having performed the appropriate tests previously and referred her to a dermatologist for a second opinion. The GP continues to reassure her that she doesn't have cancer. Despite the reassurance she remains anxious that she has skin cancer and continues to attend the GP surgery requesting further investigations.

(g) Hypochondriacal disorder

2 A 25-year-old woman presents to the clinic with a 3-month history of angry outbursts and feeling fearful and on edge all the time. She was involved in a road traffic accident 6 months ago and finds herself reliving the accident over and over again.

(h) PTSD

3   A 45-year-old woman is accompanied to the clinic by her sister. She has not left her house alone for the past 9 months. She describes heightened anxiety when leaving the house alone and had experienced two episodes of panic while in a local shop a year ago. She describes being afraid of not being able to find an exit when in public. She denies having had any further episodes of panic since that time.

   (d) Agoraphobia

CHAPTER 4

Alcohol and substance misuse disorders

MCQs

1 A 40-year-old woman is referred to the out-patient clinic by her GP. She recently lost her job because she arrived at work intoxicated. Her GP informed her 4 months ago that she has early signs of liver damage due to alcohol use. Her GP has requested that an assessment be made for an alcohol misuse problem and that appropriate treatment be offered. All the following are features of alcohol dependence syndrome as defined by ICD-10, except:

   (a) Compulsion to use alcohol
   (b) Tolerance to effects of alcohol
   (c) Court charge for driving while intoxicated
   (d) Withdrawal symptoms
   (e) Continued use despite physical harm due to alcohol use

2 A 35-year-old man with a long history of alcohol use attends the emergency department reporting high levels of anxiety, insomnia, nausea and a loss of appetite. On examination he is sweaty, with sinus tachycardia of 120 beats/min and evidence of a bilateral tremor. He reports hearing noises that others are not aware of. He reportedly had a 'fit' in the emergency department waiting area. He stopped drinking alcohol 20 h previously. A diagnosis of alcohol withdrawal is made. Which of the following would be the most appropriate treatment option:

   (a) Chlordiazepoxide
   (b) Sodium valproate
   (c) Olanzapine
   (d) Disulfiram
   (e) Propranolol

3   A 45-year-old woman attends an out-patient clinic having recently been discharged from a drug and alcohol rehabilitation centre. She is requesting medication that will aid her abstinence from alcohol. Which of the following medications is a recognised prophylactic treatment used in alcohol dependence syndrome?

(a)   Sodium valproate
(b)   Haloperidol
(c)   Diazepam
(d)   Naloxone
(e)   Disulfiram

4   A 60-year-old homeless man is brought to the emergency department by ambulance. He has a history of alcohol dependence syndrome. He is confused and agitated. He complains of double vision and he needs support while walking because of a disturbed gait. The most appropriate treatment is:

(a)   Intravenous diazepam
(b)   Intravenous thiamine
(c)   Intravenous acetylcysteine
(d)   Intravenous glucose
(e)   Intravenous gentamicin

5   You have been asked to assess a 50-year-old woman who was admitted 3 days ago to an orthopaedic ward for an elective knee arthroscopy and cartilage repair. Over the past 6 h she has become increasingly agitated. You are informed that she has a history of alcohol dependence syndrome. You suspect that she might be exhibiting features of delirium tremens. All the following features are associated with delirium tremens, except:

(a)   Autonomic instability
(b)   Visual hallucinations
(c)   Seizures
(d)   Marked tremor
(e)   Disorientation

6   A 40-year-old man attends the clinic with evidence of alcohol withdrawal symptoms. He has a history of alcohol dependence syndrome. After assessing the man, you advise that medication for his alcohol withdrawal syndrome is required. Which of the following features would indicate that medical detoxification should occur in a hospital rather than in an out-patient setting?

(a)   History of severe alcohol dependence
(b)   3 days post alcohol discontinuation with mild withdrawal symptoms evident
(c)   Experiencing social difficulties
(d)   No previous detoxification under medical supervision
(e)   History of prior successful, community-based detoxification

7   A 24-year-old woman is reviewed at the clinic. She informs you that her father has an alcohol addiction and enquires about safe drinking limits during the consultation. How many units of alcohol make up a recognised weekly safe drinking limit for women?

(a)   10 units
(b)   14 units
(c)   21 units
(d)   35 units
(e)   50 units

8   You are asked to review a 55-year-old woman in the emergency department who has a history of alcohol dependence syndrome. She is disorientated. A consultation has been requested to assess for Wernicke's encephalopathy. Which of the following features wouldn't you expect to find in Wernicke's encephalopathy?

(a)   Nystagmus
(b)   Ophthalmoplegia
(c)   Lateral rectus muscle palsy
(d)   Ataxia
(e)   Confabulation

9   A 20-year-old university student attends the clinic reporting a 1-year history of daily use of legal highs. She has recently experienced some mild paranoia on withdrawal from the use of mephedrone. Which class of drugs does mephedrone most closely resemble in its effect on users?

(a)   Amphetamines
(b)   Heroin/opioids
(c)   Cannabinoids
(d)   Hallucinogens/LSD
(e)   Methadone

10 A 24-year-old woman attends the emergency department reporting agitation. She has a history of polysubstance use. She reports insomnia for 24 h and restlessness and anxiety that has worsened over the last 12 h. On examination, the following signs are noted: watering eyes, profuse nasal secretions, sweating, shivering, dilated pupils, a pulse of 110/min and an inability to sit still. Which of the following is the most probable cause of this woman's presentation?

(a)   Heroin withdrawal
(b)   Amphetamine intoxication
(c)   Alcohol withdrawal
(d)   Cannabis intoxication
(e)   Cocaine withdrawal

11 A 24-year-old man is attending the clinic 4 weeks after discharge from hospital, having been diagnosed with a first episode of schizophrenia. You wish to discuss with him the effect cannabis might have had on him developing schizophrenia. Which of the following is true regarding the association between cannabis and schizophrenia?

   (a) Cannabis use at 26 years of age is associated with an increased risk for the development of schizophrenia compared with a younger age of cannabis use
   (b) Cannabis is associated with a 100-fold increased risk of developing schizophrenia
   (c) The majority of people who smoke cannabis will develop schizophrenia
   (d) Heavy cannabis use before 15 years of age is associated with an increased risk of schizophrenia
   (e) Cannabis use might protect against the onset of hallucinations

12 A 26-year-old male is brought to the emergency department by ambulance. He was found on the roadside by a passerby. He is unconscious and has evidence of respiratory depression, pinpoint pupils and is cold to the touch. Which of the following substances is he most likely to have had an overdose of?

   (a) Alcohol
   (b) Mephedrone
   (c) Cocaine
   (d) Benzodiazepine
   (e) Heroin

13 A 38-year-old woman has presented to the clinic reporting low mood and anxiety, ongoing for 1 month. She has a history of alcohol dependence syndrome and has been drinking alcohol on a daily basis for at least 3 months. In relation to depression and active alcohol dependence, which of the following is true?

   (a) It is appropriate to initiate an SSRI pre-detoxification as an antidepressant therapy
   (b) The patient needs to be admitted to hospital for an in-patient detoxification
   (c) The patient should be diagnosed with a depressive disorder
   (d) Most depressive and anxiety symptoms occurring pre-detoxification will not persist for greater than one month post alcohol abstinence
   (e) The presence of depression or anxiety increases the risk of seizures during alcohol withdrawal

14 A 30-year-old man attends the psychology assessment clinic. He has been referred for psychological therapy to aid him in remaining abstinent from alcohol and illicit substances. He has been abstinent from alcohol, ecstasy and heroin for 1 month. He smoked a cannabis joint with a friend yesterday and is worried that he might relapse completely and begin using alcohol and heroin again. All the following are forms of psychotherapy used in the treatment of alcohol/substance dependence, except:

(a) Methadone maintenance therapy
(b) Motivational interviewing
(c) Contingency management
(d) 12-step programmes
(e) Relapse prevention techniques

15 A 30-year-old woman with a history of recurrent depressive disorder attends the clinic to seek advice on treatment for smoking cessation. Her depression has been in remission for the past 12 months and she hasn't been treated with antidepressant medication for the past 6 months. All the following are recommended and licensed nicotine replacement therapies (as of 2015), except:

(a) Bupropion
(b) Nicotine patches
(c) Varenicline
(d) Nicotine gum
(e) Electronic cigarettes

EMI questions

Substance misuse treatments

Options:
(a) Sodium valproate
(b) Chlordiazepoxide
(c) Naloxone
(d) Cognitive–behavioural therapy
(e) Fluoxetine
(f) Quetiapine
(g) Disulfiram
(h) Admission to a specialist alcohol treatment centre

Select an intervention that would be recommended for each of the following clinical scenarios.

1 A 45-year-old man presents to the emergency department with a history of a seizure 3 h ago. Prior to this seizure, he reports experiencing anxiety, insomnia, palpitations and sweating. He had been drinking heavily for 2 weeks until 20 h ago.

2 A 40-year-old father of two presents to the psychiatry clinic. He has a 10-year history of alcohol dependence and has failed multiple out-patient treatment programmes. He was discharged from hospital yesterday after an admission for medical treatment of alcohol withdrawal and hasn't had a drink since that time. He states that he wants to stop drinking.

3 A 34-year-old is referred to the addictions clinic by his GP. He had recently relapsed with alcohol use, following a period of abstinence supported by attending a 12-step Alcoholics Anonymous programme. He has been abstinent for the past week and wishes to access support to reduce his risk of drinking in the community and is seeking medical intervention. He is physically well at present.

Illicit substance use

Options:

    (a)   Heroin
    (b)   LSD
    (c)   Amphetamines
    (d)   Alcohol
    (e)   Ecstasy
    (f)   Khat
    (g)   Mephedrone
    (h)   Cannabis

Select the substance that is most likely to have been consumed in the following clinical scenarios.

1 A 65-year-old woman presents to the emergency department in a confused and agitated state. She has gait imbalance and complains of double vision.

2 An 18-year-old college student attends the emergency department with acute anxiety. There is evidence of visual hallucinations, heightened colour sensitivity, and derealisation and depersonalisation phenomena. He reports that he took a drug 6 h ago and that he initially felt relaxed, but that anxiety has increased with the occurrence of the described symptoms.

3 A 28-year-old man is brought to the emergency department by ambulance. He reports that he is a regular drug user and that he last took a drug 2 h ago. He reports palpitations, dry mouth and a sensation of insects crawling under his skin. He presents with agitation, lability of mood, tachycardia and dilated pupils.

MCQ answers

1   A 40-year-old woman is referred to the out-patient clinic by her GP. She recently lost her job because she arrived at work intoxicated. Her GP informed her 4 months ago that she has early signs of liver damage due to alcohol use. Her GP has requested that an assessment be made for an alcohol misuse problem and that appropriate treatment be offered. All the following are features of alcohol dependence syndrome as defined by ICD-10, except:

(a)   Compulsion to use alcohol
(b)   Tolerance to effects of alcohol
(c)   **Court charge for driving while intoxicated**
(d)   Withdrawal symptoms
(e)   Continued use despite physical harm due to alcohol use

Alcohol dependence syndrome is a cluster of physiological, behavioural, and cognitive phenomena in which the use of alcohol takes on a much higher priority for a person than behaviours that once had greater value. ICD-10 does not specify social or legal consequences of alcohol use as a criterion for alcohol dependence syndrome. DSM-5 specifies recurrent social problems due to alcohol use as a criterion for its alcohol use disorder (which replaces the previous diagnostic dichotomy of alcohol abuse and alcohol dependence syndrome in DSM-IV). The ICD-10 harmful use of alcohol category requires evidence that substance use is responsible for physical or psychological harm. See APA (2013) and WHO (1992).

2   A 35-year-old man with a long history of alcohol use attends the emergency department reporting high levels of anxiety, insomnia, nausea and a loss of appetite. On examination he is sweaty, with sinus tachycardia of 120 beats/min and evidence of a bilateral tremor. He reports hearing noises that others are not aware of. He reportedly had a 'fit' in the emergency department waiting area. He stopped drinking alcohol 20h previously. A diagnosis of alcohol withdrawal is made. Which of the following would be the most appropriate treatment option:

(a)   **Chlordiazepoxide**
(b)   Sodium valproate
(c)   Olanzapine
(d)   Disulfiram
(e)   Propranolol

Benzodiazepines remain the mainstay of treatment for alcohol withdrawal syndromes. Longer-acting benzodiazepines such as chlordiazepoxide or diazepam are the preferred medications, offering smoother management of the withdrawal period because of their longer duration of action. In patients with evidence of liver impairment, shorter-acting benzodiazepines such as oxazepam or lorazepam should be used to avoid accumulation of benzodiazepines. Benzodiazepines are generally prescribed for 5 days to treat alcohol withdrawal and prevent seizures and delirium tremens, although a longer duration might be required for more severe withdrawal symptoms or dependence. See Perry (2014) and Taylor *et al* (2012).

3   A 45-year-old woman attends an outpatient clinic having recently been discharged from a drug and alcohol rehabilitation centre. She is requesting medication that will aid her abstinence from alcohol. Which of the following medications is a recognised prophylactic treatment used in alcohol dependence syndrome?

  (a)   Sodium valproate
  (b)   Haloperidol
  (c)   Diazepam
  (d)   Naloxone
  (e)   **Disulfiram**

Pharmacotherapy for the maintenance of abstinence in alcohol dependence syndrome has a poor evidence base, with few treatments proven to be highly effective. Disulfiram has been used to treat alcohol-use disorders for over half a century.

Disulfiram causes inhibition of alcohol dehydrogenase and concomitant accumulation of acetaldehyde, which produces an aversive reaction when combined with alcohol. Individuals who use alcohol while taking disulfiram can experience a range of adverse effects, including nausea, vomiting, head, neck and chest flushing, throbbing headaches, vertigo, ataxia, weakness, diaphoresis, tachycardia, orthostatic hypotension and palpitations. Disulfiram works by aversive conditioning, rather than a direct effect on alcohol craving.

Naloxone is a pure opioid antagonist used in opioid toxicity to reverse the effects of opioid intoxication. (Naltrexone, which should not be confused with naloxone, is an opioid-receptor antagonist used to aid the maintenance of abstinence in alcohol dependence syndrome.) See Taylor *et al* (2012).

4   A 60-year-old homeless man is brought to the emergency department by ambulance. He has a history of alcohol dependence syndrome. He is confused and agitated. He complains of double vision and he needs support while walking because of a disturbed gait. The most appropriate treatment is:

  (a)   Intravenous diazepam
  (b)   **Intravenous thiamine**
  (c)   Intravenous acetylcysteine
  (d)   Intravenous glucose
  (e)   Intravenous gentamicin

This man is presenting with features of Wernicke's encephalopathy (see question 8). Wernicke's encephalopathy is a medical emergency. Untreated, it leads to death in up to 20% of cases and to Korsakoff's syndrome in 85% of survivors. Up to 25% of the people with Korsakoff's syndrome will require long-term institutionalisation. When Wernicke's encephalopathy is suspected, treatment with high-dose parenteral thiamine should be given promptly to offset the risk of death and the development of Korsakoff's syndrome. See Greenberg (2001) and Taylor *et al* (2012).

5   You have been asked to assess a 50-year-old woman who was admitted 3 days ago
     to an orthopaedic ward for an elective knee arthroscopy and cartilage repair. Over
     the past 6h she has become increasingly agitated. You are informed that she has a
     history of alcohol dependence syndrome. You suspect that she might be exhibiting
     features of delirium tremens. All the following features are associated with delirium
     tremens, except:
     (a)   Autonomic instability
     (b)   Visual hallucinations
     (c)   **Seizures**
     (d)   Marked tremor
     (e)   Disorientation

Delirium tremens is the most serious acute complication of alcohol
withdrawal. It is the result of under-treatment or lack of treatment of
alcohol withdrawal symptoms. Delirium tremens occurs in approximately
5% of patients hospitalised for alcohol withdrawal syndrome and the
mortality rate is 5–15%. Onset is typically 3–5 days after the last drink.
Alcohol-withdrawal syndrome with delirium is defined in ICD-10 as
delirium accompanied by autonomic hyperactivity, visual and auditory
hallucinations, clouding of consciousness, agitation and tremor. Seizures
due to alcohol withdrawal generally occur within 24h of discontinuation of
drinking, but are not part of the criteria for delirium tremens.

Alcohol withdrawal symptoms appear within hours of the last drink and
peak 24–48h after the last drink. Delirium tremens peaks 72–96h after the
last drink. See Perry (2014) and Taylor *et al* (2012).

6   A 40-year-old man attends the clinic with evidence of alcohol withdrawal symptoms.
     He has a history of alcohol dependence syndrome. After assessing the man, you
     advise that medication for his alcohol withdrawal syndrome is required. Which of
     the following features would indicate that medical detoxification should occur in a
     hospital rather than in an out-patient setting?
     (a)   **History of severe alcohol dependence**
     (b)   3 days post alcohol discontinuation with mild withdrawal symptoms evident
     (c)   Experiencing social difficulties
     (d)   No previous detoxification under medical supervision
     (e)   History of prior successful, community-based detoxification

Features in a patient's history that indicate that in-patient medical
detoxification is required include the following:
▶ severity of prior episodes of alcohol withdrawal symptoms, including
  detoxification, seizures, or delirium tremens
▶ older age
▶ moderate to severe withdrawal symptoms at baseline
▶ concomitant medical or surgical illness (e.g. trauma, infections, sepsis,
  liver disease)

- severity of dependence (quantity, frequency, duration of dependence)
- abnormal liver function (e.g. elevated aspartate aminotransferase)
- time since last drink (onset of delirium tremens is generally 3–5 days after the last drink)
- prior benzodiazepine use/misuse (as this might mean that the patient will be benzodiazepine tolerant and requiring a higher dose of benzodiazepines for medical detoxification) or concurrent substance misuse (polydrug use)
- history of failed community detoxification.

See Taylor *et al* (2012).

7   A 24-year-old woman is reviewed at the clinic. She informs you that her father has an alcohol addiction and enquires about safe drinking limits during the consultation. How many units of alcohol make up a recognised weekly safe drinking limit for women?

    (a)   10 units
    (b)   **14 units**
    (c)   21 units
    (d)   35 units
    (e)   50 units

The formula for calculating units of alcohol is as follows:

alcohol by volume (%) × volume (mL) / 1000 = units

For example, a pint of 4% beer of 568 mL in volume contains 4 × 568/1000 units of alcohol, or 2.27 units.

The recommended safe drinking limit for women is 14 units of alcohol per week, no more than 3 units in any given day, and at least 2 alcohol-free days a week. For women, drinking 14–35 units of alcohol per week is considered hazardous drinking and drinking more than 35 units of alcohol per week is considered harmful drinking. See NICE (2011*a*).

8   You are asked to review a 55-year-old woman in the emergency department who has a history of alcohol dependence syndrome. She is disorientated. A consultation has been requested to assess for Wernicke's encephalopathy. Which of the following features wouldn't you expect to find in Wernicke's encephalopathy?

    (a)   Nystagmus
    (b)   Ophthalmoplegia
    (c)   Lateral rectus muscle palsy
    (d)   Ataxia
    (e)   **Confabulation**

Wernicke's encephalopathy is characterised by a tetrad of symptoms: acute confusional state, ataxia, nystagmus and ophthalmoplegia (most commonly sixth nerve palsy with paralysis of the lateral rectus muscle and of conjugate gaze). Associated features include tachycardia and peripheral neuropathy. Wernicke's encephalopathy represents the acute neuropsychiatric reaction and the related condition Korsakoff's syndrome represents the residual and, sometimes, permanent defect. If Wernicke's encephalopathy goes untreated, there is a 15–20% mortality rate, and 85% of cases will develop Korsakoff's syndrome. This is residual impairment in the ability to form new memories and is often permanent. Confabulation, which is seen in Korsakoff's syndrome, is fabrication of ideas and information that are not consistent with reality (i.e. 'filling in the blanks' for periods of amnesia). Both Wernicke's encephalopathy and Korsakoff's syndrome are caused by thiamine (vitamin B1) deficiency and most often occur secondary to alcohol misuse disorders. See Greenberg & Lee (2001).

9 A 20-year-old university student attends the clinic reporting a 1-year history of daily use of legal highs. She has recently experienced some mild paranoia on withdrawal from the use of mephedrone. Which class of drugs does mephedrone most closely resemble in its effect on users?

   (a) **Amphetamines**
   (b) Heroin/opioids
   (c) Cannabinoids
   (d) Hallucinogens/LSD
   (e) Methadone

'Legal highs' is a term used to describe a range of psychoactive substances (some of which are designed to mimic the effects of illicit drugs). They are often legal to begin with, as they represent novel psychoactive substances. As in the case of mephedrone (4-methylmethcathinone), which was criminalised in 2010 in the UK, a reclassification from legal to illegal can often occur as problems with their use emerge. Mephedrone is a cathinone, which users describe as having an effect similar to amphetamines or ecstasy. It acts as a psycho-stimulant. The estimated prevalence of the use of mephedrone in the UK in those 16–24 years of age is 2–5%.

Similarly, synthetic cannabinoids found in substances like 'spice' probably evoke a physiologic response similar to tetrahydrocannabinol (THC). The use of legal highs has been reported in as many as 13% of individuals with a psychiatric illness and has been associated with a deleterious effect on the mental state of those with a mental illness, especially those with psychosis. See Lally *et al* (2013).

10 A 24-year-old woman attends the emergency department reporting agitation. She has a history of polysubstance use. She reports insomnia for 24 h and restlessness and anxiety that has worsened over the last 12 h. On examination, the following signs are noted: watering eyes, profuse nasal secretions, sweating, shivering, dilated pupils, a pulse of 110/min and an inability to sit still. Which of the following is the most probable cause of this woman's presentation?

    (a)   **Heroin withdrawal**
    (b)   Amphetamine intoxication
    (c)   Alcohol withdrawal
    (d)   Cannabis intoxication
    (e)   Cocaine withdrawal

Physical symptoms of opioid withdrawal include myalgia, yawning, perspiration, lacrimation, rhinitis, nausea, restlessness/agitation and heart rate > 100 beats/min. Psychological symptoms include anxiety, irritability, fatigue and insomnia. Signs and symptoms usually begin 2–3 half-lives after the last opioid dose: 36–48 h for long half-life opioids such as methadone, and 6–12 h for short half-life opioids such as heroin and morphine. After cessation of heroin, symptoms reach peak intensity within 2–4 days, with most of the obvious physical withdrawal signs no longer observable after 7 days. The duration of methadone withdrawal is longer (5–21 days). Opioid withdrawal syndrome is rarely life-threatening. See Kleber (2007).

11 A 24-year-old man is attending the clinic 4 weeks after discharge from hospital, having been diagnosed with a first episode of schizophrenia. You wish to discuss with him the effect cannabis might have had on him developing schizophrenia. Which of the following is true regarding the association between cannabis and schizophrenia?

    (a)   Cannabis use at 26 years of age is associated with an increased risk for the development of schizophrenia compared with a younger age of cannabis use
    (b)   Cannabis is associated with a 100-fold increased risk of developing schizophrenia
    (c)   The majority of people who smoke cannabis will develop schizophrenia
    (d)   **Heavy cannabis use before 15 years of age is associated with an increased risk of schizophrenia**
    (e)   Cannabis use might protect against the onset of hallucinations

Accumulating evidence from longitudinal epidemiologic studies suggests that cannabis use might increase the risk of schizophrenia and psychosis. However, rather than serving as a component cause of the disorder, cannabis represents one of a constellation of complex factors that can hasten the development of psychotic symptoms, while neither necessary for their development nor sufficient to do so alone. Those using cannabis before 15 years of age are 3.4 times more likely than controls to meet diagnostic criteria for schizophreniform disorder at 26 years of age, and those who smoked more cannabis more frequently are at a higher risk, demonstrating a dose–response effect. Meta-analyses and systematic reviews have consistently found a two-fold greater risk for psychosis among cannabis users. See Arseneault et al (2014) and Moore et al (2007).

12 A 26-year-old male is brought to the emergency department by ambulance. He was found on the roadside by a passerby. He is unconscious and has evidence of respiratory depression, pinpoint pupils and is cold to the touch. Which of the following substances is he most likely to have had an overdose of?

(a) Alcohol
(b) Mephedrone
(c) Cocaine
(d) Benzodiazepine
(e) **Heroin**

This man has presented with features of an opioid/heroin overdose. Death can occur from respiratory depression. Patients should be managed with cardiopulmonary resuscitation protocol as required. Naloxone is a pure opioid antagonist that can be administered intramuscularly to reverse the effects of the overdose. Naloxone acts within 2–8 min and has duration of action of 30–60 min, meaning that symptoms of an opioid overdose might return. Naloxone might have to be repeated at intervals and the patient should be monitored for several hours afterwards. See Taylor *et al* (2012).

13 A 38-year-old woman has presented to the clinic reporting low mood and anxiety, ongoing for 1 month. She has a history of alcohol dependence syndrome and has been drinking alcohol on a daily basis for at least 3 months. In relation to depression and active alcohol dependence, which of the following is true?

(a) It is appropriate to initiate an SSRI pre-detoxification as an antidepressant therapy
(b) The patient needs to be admitted to hospital for an in-patient detoxification
(c) The patient should be diagnosed with a depressive disorder
(d) **Most depressive and anxiety symptoms occurring pre-detoxification will not persist for greater than one month post alcohol abstinence**
(e) The presence of depression or anxiety increases the risk of seizures during alcohol withdrawal

In persons with comorbid mood and substance use disorders, the ICD-10 and DSM-5 diagnostic criteria indicate that the mood disorder is primary if it is not due to the effects of alcohol or drugs. But if the mood disorder arises during the course of alcohol or drug use, it should be considered secondary to the alcohol or substance use. For the majority of people who can remain abstinent from alcohol, their mood and anxiety symptoms will improve within one month. However, for those in whom depression or anxiety persist, pharmacotherapy along with psychotherapy should be initiated to treat the affective disorder. See Brown *et al* (1995).

14 A 30-year-old man attends the psychology assessment clinic. He has been referred for psychological therapy to aid him in remaining abstinent from alcohol and illicit substances. He has been abstinent from alcohol, ecstasy and heroin for 1 month. He smoked a cannabis joint with a friend yesterday and is worried that he might relapse completely and begin using alcohol and heroin again. All the following are forms of psychotherapy used in the treatment of alcohol/substance dependence, except:

    (a)   **Methadone maintenance therapy**
    (b)   Motivational interviewing
    (c)   Contingency management
    (d)   12-step programmes
    (e)   Relapse prevention techniques

Methadone maintenance therapy is a pharmacotherapy used in the treatment of heroin dependence, with the aim of reducing heroin compulsion and use and inducing an associated decrease in harmful lifestyle choices. Methadone is a long-acting synthetic opioid agonist, which can be dosed once daily.

The other four items are all psychotherapeutic interventions for alcohol/substance dependence. The 12-step programmes refers to group programmes such as Alcoholics Anonymous, which is voluntary and in which group support and self-growth are pivotal features supporting an individual in maintaining abstinence. Underpinning motivational interviewing is the 'stages of change' model (pre-contemplation, contemplation, preparation, action, maintenance, relapse). With contingency management strategies, abstinence leads to the individual gaining certain rewards, such as financial or employment benefits. See NICE (2007, 2011a).

15 A 30-year-old woman with a history of recurrent depressive disorder attends the clinic to seek advice on treatment for smoking cessation. Her depression has been in remission for the past 12 months and she hasn't been treated with antidepressant medication for the past 6 months. All the following are recommended and licensed nicotine replacement therapies (as of 2015), except:

    (a)   Bupropion
    (b)   Nicotine patches
    (c)   Varenicline
    (d)   Nicotine gum
    (e)   **Electronic cigarettes**

Electronic cigarettes are not a licensed treatment for smoking cessation. They cannot be prescribed for this specific purpose, through many people use them of their own volition to aid smoking cessation. Nicotine patches, gum, inhalator, lozenges and nasal sprays can all be prescribed as monotherapy for smoking cessation or as combinations for those with evidence of severe nicotine dependence. Bupropion and varenicline are medications licensed for use in smoking cessation. See Taylor et al (2012).

EMI answers

Substance misuse treatments

Options:

(a)   Sodium valproate
(b)   Chlordiazepoxide
(c)   Naloxone
(d)   Cognitive–behavioural therapy
(e)   Fluoxetine
(f)   Quetiapine
(g)   Disulfiram
(h)   Admission to a specialist alcohol treatment centre

Select an intervention that would be recommended for each of the following clinical scenarios.

1   A 45-year-old man presents to the emergency department with a history of a seizure 3 h ago. Prior to this seizure, he reports experiencing anxiety, insomnia, palpitations and sweating. He had been drinking heavily for 2 weeks until 20 h ago.

(b) Chlordiazepoxide

2   A 40-year-old father of two presents to the psychiatry clinic. He has a 10-year history of alcohol dependence and has failed multiple out-patient treatment programmes. He was discharged from hospital yesterday after an admission for medical treatment of alcohol withdrawal and hasn't had a drink since that time. He states that he wants to stop drinking.

(h) Admission to a specialist alcohol treatment centre

3   A 34-year-old is referred to the addictions clinic by his GP. He had recently relapsed with alcohol use, following a period of abstinence supported by attending a 12-step Alcoholics Anonymous programme. He has been abstinent for the past week and wishes to access support to reduce his risk of drinking in the community and is seeking medical intervention. He is physically well at present.

(g) Disulfiram

Illicit substance use

Options:

(a)   Heroin
(b)   LSD
(c)   Amphetamines
(d)   Alcohol
(e)   Ecstasy
(f)   Khat
(g)   Mephedrone
(h)   Cannabis

Select the substance that is most likely to have been consumed in the following clinical scenarios.

1 A 65-year-old woman presents to the emergency department in a confused and agitated state. She has gait imbalance and complains of double vision.

   (d) Alcohol

2 An 18-year-old college student attends the emergency department with acute anxiety. There is evidence of visual hallucinations, heightened colour sensitivity, and derealisation and depersonalisation phenomena. He reports that he took a drug 6 h ago and that he initially felt relaxed, but that anxiety has increased with the occurrence of the described symptoms.

   (b) LSD

3 A 28-year-old man is brought to the emergency department by ambulance. He reports that he is a regular drug user and that he last took a drug 2 h ago. He reports palpitations, dry mouth and a sensation of insects crawling under his skin. He presents with agitation, lability of mood, tachycardia and dilated pupils.

   (c) Amphetamines

CHAPTER 5

Old age psychiatry and organic disorders

MCQs

1   A 73-year-old woman is assessed at a memory clinic. She has an MMSE score of 18, reduced from 23 a year ago. What does this finding tell you?
    (a)   She has Alzheimer's disease
    (b)   She has had a stroke
    (c)   She has mild cognitive impairment
    (d)   Her cognitive function is declining
    (e)   She has Parkinson's disease

2   A 66-year-old man is referred to your clinic. His wife attends with him and tells you that he has been forgetful of late. He often forgets where he leaves his keys and yesterday he forgot about his appointment with you. He has been repeating questions and finding it difficult to express himself and has been more irritable than usual. He scores 23/30 on the MMSE. What diagnosis would you be most concerned about at this stage?
    (a)   Delirium
    (b)   Frontotemporal dementia
    (c)   Lewy body dementia
    (d)   Alzheimer's disease
    (e)   Late-onset schizophrenia

3   You are asked to review an 82-year-old man with Alzheimer's disease in his care home. He does not recognise his family members and his MMSE score is 15. Which of the following drugs is he most likely to be on?
    (a)   Donepezil
    (b)   Haloperidol
    (c)   Olanzapine
    (d)   Memantine
    (e)   Procyclidine

4   A 61-year-old man with hypertension, diabetes mellitus and ischaemic heart disease is referred to your clinic. He has a relatively rapid onset of difficulty in planning his daily activities, being more irritable than usual and forgetting events he has planned. For the next 2 years, he functions largely at the same level before he has a stroke and experiences further decline in cognitive performance. What is the most likely diagnosis here?

   (a)   Alzheimer's disease
   (b)   Frontotemporal dementia
   (c)   Lewy body dementia
   (d)   Pseudodementia
   (e)   Vascular dementia

5   A 67-year-old woman presents to the emergency department reporting seeing 'little red animals all around'. Her daughter, who accompanies her, tells you that she was speaking clearly and sensibly earlier in the day and has been describing these animals in detail for some weeks. She has been experiencing memory difficulties for many months that fluctuate in severity. On examination you find that she has stiffness and resting tremor in her upper limbs. Her daughter tells you that this symptom has emerged only in recent weeks. What is her probable diagnosis?

   (a)   Parkinson's disease
   (b)   Lewy body dementia
   (c)   Huntington's disease
   (d)   Alzheimer's disease
   (e)   Delirium tremens

6   A 54-year-old man is referred by his GP because of behavioural change over the past 6 months. His wife has noticed that he has been more irritable than usual, with outbursts of verbal aggression towards her that are completely out of character. He is less affectionate towards her and colder with people generally. He has become involved in rows with his neighbours, which never happened before. He has also been making inappropriate and lewd jokes and using made-up words, sometimes in public. He does not think that there is anything wrong with him. His MMSE score is 25. What is the most likely cause of his altered behaviour?

   (a)   Lewy body dementia
   (b)   Alzheimer's disease
   (c)   Vascular dementia
   (d)   Frontotemporal dementia
   (e)   Depression

7   A 34-year-old man is referred to your out-patient clinic. He complains of low mood over the past 6 months. He also describes occasional difficulty in reading and writing and dressing himself. On full examination, he has difficulty in naming parts of objects, such as the second hand on your watch. Recently, he has been getting headaches. Where is the probable pathology?

   (a)   Cerebellum
   (b)   Parietal lobe
   (c)   Temporal lobe
   (d)   Frontal lobe
   (e)   Corpus callosum

8   A 72-year-old woman is assessed at your clinic. Her husband is worried about her as she has 'not been herself' and has lost interest in things. She is not sleeping and has lost weight. She has been having a lot of physical health problems, including leg pain and abdominal cramps, and she is convinced she has cancer, although her GP has found nothing wrong. She denies feeling sad or upset. On cognitive assessment, she scores poorly, but this is mainly because she answers 'don't know' to most questions, even straightforward ones. What do you think her diagnosis is?

   (a)   Dementia
   (b)   Psychosis
   (c)   Depression
   (d)   Delirium
   (e)   No diagnosis

9   A 78-year-old man with severe depressive illness is referred to your clinic and you start him on an antidepressant. A few weeks later, his GP writes to you informing you that he is stopping the antidepressant as it has resulted in hyponatraemia. What medication most likely to be the offending agent?

   (a)   Amitriptyline
   (b)   Citalopram
   (c)   Mirtazapine
   (d)   Duloxetine
   (e)   Trazadone

10 A 23-year-old is assessed in the emergency department. He complains of a feeling of intense fear, associated with an odd sensation of having been in the exact same situation before. He describes having experienced an intense smell of rotting vegetables. All these sensations passed after a period of 1–2 min but for a time after he felt strange and then exhausted. The treating consultant suggests he might have had a seizure. Which type of seizure is he most likely to have had?

(a) Tonic–clonic seizure
(b) Absence seizure
(c) Atonic seizure
(d) Temporal lobe epilepsy seizure
(e) Non-epileptiform seizure

11 Which two types of psychiatric disorder are most common in patients with epilepsy?

(a) Depression and anxiety
(b) Depression and psychosis
(c) Psychosis and anxiety
(d) OCD and depression
(e) OCD and psychosis

12 A 71-year-old woman with pneumonia becomes increasingly agitated throughout the course of an evening. She does not have a diagnosis of dementia but, during assessment, it is difficult to maintain her attention and she cannot tell you what day or date it is or where she is. She seems distracted and describes seeing insects climbing on the wall, although there are none there. What is this woman's probable diagnosis?

(a) Schizophrenia
(b) Depression
(c) New-onset Alzheimer's disease
(d) Parkinson's disease
(e) Delirium

13 A 36-year-old man is involved in a road traffic accident. He smashes his head against the window and is rendered unconscious. He loses consciousness for several minutes but then begins to recover. He is taken to hospital to be assessed. Which type of memory loss is most common in such injuries?

(a) Retrograde memory loss
(b) Procedural memory loss
(c) Anterograde memory loss
(d) Semantic memory loss
(e) Working memory loss

14 A 17-year-old boy is brought to hospital after collapsing on the rugby field following a collision. Which investigation will be most useful in assessing injury to his brain?

(a) Skull X-ray
(b) Magnetic resonance imaging (MRI) spectroscopy of the brain
(c) Electroencephalogram
(d) Positron emission tomography (PET)
(e) Computed tomography (CT) of the brain

15 A 37-year-old woman presents reporting feeling anxious, hyperactive and irritable most of the time for the past 2 months. She also complains of weight loss (despite an increased appetite), intolerance to heat, hair loss, muscle aches, weakness, fatigue and intermittent diarrhoea. Which of the following endocrine conditions is most likely to explain her symptoms?

(a) Diabetes mellitus
(b) Addison's disease
(c) Phaeochromocytoma
(d) Diabetes insipidus
(e) Hyperthyroidism

16 A 68-year-old man is referred to your clinic. He holds the fixed belief that his neighbours are entering his house by passing through the walls. He says he can hear their voices in his living room even when he cannot see them there. He does not have first-rank symptoms of schizophrenia. He does not have low or elevated mood. He scores 30/30 on the MMSE, is orientated to time, place and person and does not have visual hallucinations. What is his most likely diagnosis?

(a) Alzheimer's disease
(b) Depression
(c) Mania
(d) Late-onset schizophrenia
(e) Delirium

EMI questions

Cognitive assessment

Options:

    (a) MMSE
    (b) Addenbrooke's Cognitive Examination
    (c) Frontal lobe battery
    (d) Astereognosis and agraphesthesia
    (e) Spelling WORLD backwards
    (f) Registration and recall
    (g) Difficulty naming dates of World War II
    (h) Intersecting pentagons

Match the items above with the items below. (Each option is used once only.)

1   A screening and monitoring test for cognitive impairment

2   A test of visuospatial skills

3   Tested using 'apple, penny, table' in MMSE

4   Indicates semantic memory impairment

5   Indicates parietal lobe impairment

6   Tests language skills in more detail than MMSE

7   Includes Luria test and 'go/no-go' test

8   Test of attention

Medications in old age psychiatry

Options:

    (a) Donepezil
    (b) Mirtazapine
    (c) Second-generation antipsychotics
    (d) Haloperidol
    (e) Galantamine
    (f) SNRIs
    (g) SSRIs

Match the items above with the answers below. (More than one answer may be given for each item below.)

1   Acetylcholinesterase inhibitors used in dementia (select two options)

2   Particular caution advised in the elderly because of risk of cerebrovascular adverse events (select one option)

3   First-line antidepressants used in the elderly (select two options)

4   Another antidepressant used in the elderly (select one option)

Symptoms, signs and test results

Options:

(a) Jerky, random, and uncontrollable movements in a 40-year-old man
(b) Visual hallucination
(c) Fluctuating cognitive impairment
(d) Genetic test indicating autosomal dominant condition
(e) Hyperthermia and muscle rigidity
(f) Highly impaired attention on mental state exam
(g) Resting tremor and bradykinesia
(h) Agitation that is worse at night
(i) Highly elevated creatine phosphokinase

Match the items above with the answers below. (Each answer below has more than one matching item. Each item may be used more than once.)

1 Lewy body dementia (select three options)

2 Huntington's disease (select two options)

3 Neuroleptic malignant syndrome (select two options)

4 Delirium (select four options)

MCQ answers

1 A 73-year-old woman is assessed at a memory clinic. She has an MMSE score of 18, reduced from 23 a year ago. What does this finding tell you?
(a) She has Alzheimer's disease
(b) She has had a stroke
(c) She has mild cognitive impairment
(d) **Her cognitive function is declining**
(e) She has Parkinson's disease

Introduced in 1975, the MMSE is a widely used, if often misunderstood, cognitive screening tool. The MMSE is useful in screening for and tracking decline in cognitive impairment, which can be categorised using the MMSE score as mild (usually 21–26), moderate (usually 10–20) or severe (<10). The level of cognitive impairment is in turn used as a guide for when to introduce different pharmacological treatments for dementia, depending on the underlying cause (see question 3).

It should be noted that the MMSE is weighted significantly towards certain aspects of memory and attention and is relatively insensitive for frontal and subcortical impairment. The patient's educational background, age and first language also need to be considered. As with all psychometric tools, its usefulness is also dependent on the ability of the examiner to apply it in a correct and consistent manner. See Kipps & Hodges (2008) and, for further reading, Folstein *et al* (1975).

2   A 66-year-old man is referred to your clinic. His wife attends with him and tells
    you that he has been forgetful of late. He often forgets where he leaves his keys and
    yesterday he forgot about his appointment with you. He has been repeating questions
    and finding it difficult to express himself and has been more irritable than usual. He
    scores 23/30 on the MMSE. What diagnosis would you be most concerned about at
    this stage?
    (a)   Delirium
    (b)   Frontotemporal dementia
    (c)   Lewy body dementia
    (d)   **Alzheimer's disease**
    (e)   Late-onset schizophrenia

This man seems to be in the early stages of Alzheimer's disease. It is the
most common form of dementia, accounting for 60–70% of cases, and
places an enormous healthcare burden on society and carers. Advancing age
is a primary risk factor: every 5 years after the age of 65, the risk of acquiring
the disease doubles. The cause remains unknown, although is thought
to represent a combination of genetic, vascular and inflammatory risk
factors. Alzheimer's disease results in neuronal loss, chiefly in the cortex,
resulting in gross atrophy of the affected regions, including degeneration
in the temporal lobe and parietal lobe, and parts of the frontal cortex and
cingulate gyrus. The key histopathological findings are amyloid plaques and
neurofibrillary tangles.

Memory impairment is the most common presenting complaint and is
typically accompanied by a history of misplacing and losing objects. Other
changes noticeable in the early stages include word-finding difficulties
and subtle personality changes. A score of less than 27/30 on the MMSE
should further raise suspicion (see question 1). Ongoing assessment will
be required here as the diagnostic criteria are complex. See Thomas (2008)
and, for further reading, Alzheimer's Association (n.d., 2013) and Wenk
(2003).

3   You are asked to review an 82-year-old man with Alzheimer's disease in his care
    home. He does not recognise his family members and his MMSE score is 15. Which
    of the following drugs is he most likely to be on?
    (a)   **Donepezil**
    (b)   Haloperidol
    (c)   Olanzapine
    (d)   Memantine
    (e)   Procyclidine

As Alzheimer's disease progresses, acetylcholine decreases in areas
of the brain associated with amyloid deposition. Acetylcholinesterase
inhibitors are drugs that inhibit acetylcholinesterase from breaking down
acetylcholine, thereby increasing both the level and duration of action of
acetylcholine, thus enhancing cholinergic regulation in the brain. Three
acetylcholinesterase inhibitors (donepezil, galantamine and rivastigmine)

are recommended as options for managing mild to moderate Alzheimer's disease. These drugs improve the short-term prognosis of Alzheimer's disease for the 50–60% of patients who respond to them. They are less useful in severe Alzheimer's disease, where the risks are thought to outweigh the benefits.

Memantine is a drug that modulates glutamate through the blockade of N-methyl-D-aspartate receptor channels. It is recommended as an option for people with severe Alzheimer's disease or with moderate disease who are intolerant of or have a contraindication for acetylcholinesterase inhibitors. Although often used for the treatment of specific dementia symptoms, antipsychotics should be prescribed with caution. They are associated with an increased mortality risk in this population. See NICE (2011*b*), Stewart (2008) and Thomas (2008) and, for further reading, Maust *et al* (2015) and Schneider *et al* (2011).

4 A 61-year-old man with hypertension, diabetes mellitus and ischaemic heart disease is referred to your clinic. He has a relatively rapid onset of difficulty in planning his daily activities, being more irritable than usual and forgetting events he has planned. For the next 2 years, he functions largely at the same level before he has a stroke and experiences further decline in cognitive performance. What is the most likely diagnosis here?

   (a) Alzheimer's disease
   (b) Frontotemporal dementia
   (c) Lewy body dementia
   (d) Pseudodementia
   (e) **Vascular dementia**

This man has vascular dementia. Although difficulties exist with classification and diagnosis of this condition, as a general rule, a step-wise deterioration in cognitive performance in an individual with multiple vascular risk factors is likely to have a significant vascular contribution. Impairments can result from multiple small infarcts (multi-infarct dementia) or larger infarcts, which can lead to disproportionate impairment of one brain area (e.g. parietal lobe dysfunction).

Vascular dementia is the second most common cause of dementia after Alzheimer's disease, accounting for 20–30% of cases. Many cases of vascular dementia represent mixed dementia – vascular dementia with Alzheimer's disease – and there is evidence implicating a comorbid underlying pathology for vascular dementia and Alzheimer's disease. Many cases of dementia following stroke seem to follow an Alzheimer's-disease-like clinical course without further infarction. See Stewart (2008) and, for further reading, Viswanathan *et al* (2009).

5   A 67-year-old woman presents to the emergency department reporting seeing 'little red animals all around'. Her daughter, who accompanies her, tells you that she was speaking clearly and sensibly earlier in the day and has been describing these animals in detail for some weeks. She has been experiencing memory difficulties for many months that fluctuate in severity. On examination you find that she has stiffness and resting tremor in her upper limbs. Her daughter tells you that this symptom has emerged only in recent weeks. What is her probable diagnosis?

(a)   Parkinson's disease
(b)   **Lewy body dementia**
(c)   Huntington's disease
(d)   Alzheimer's disease
(e)   Delirium tremens

Lewy body dementia (LBD; also known as dementia with Lewy bodies) is a form of dementia with the key pathological feature of Lewy bodies. These are neuronal inclusion bodies that are also found in Parkinson's disease. In LBD, these structures appear more often in the cortex, and in Parkinson's disease dementia they are usually found in subcortical structures.

Diagnosis of LBD is not straightforward, as it shares many features with other dementias, particularly Parkinson's disease and vascular dementia. However, whereas cognitive symptoms precede or are closely followed by motor symptoms in LBD, motor symptoms occur at least a year before the cognitive impairment in Parkinson's disease dementia. In this case, the patient has all three core clinical features of LBD: recurrent, well-formed visual hallucinations; fluctuating cognition with pronounced variations in attention and alertness; and spontaneous features of Parkinsonism. Diagnosis is important because antipsychotic medications, which are sometimes used to treat agitation in dementia and may be used to treat psychotic features, can lead to adverse outcomes in LBD. This is due to neuroleptic sensitivity, which can lead to irreversible Parkinsonism and autonomic dysfunction similar to neuropleptic malignant syndrome.

Although visual hallucinations and confusion occur in delirium tremens, that diagnosis does not account for the range or duration of symptoms here. See Stewart (2008) and, for further reading, McKeith *et al* (2005).

6   A 54-year-old man is referred by his GP because of behavioural change over the past 6 months. His wife has noticed that he has been more irritable than usual, with outbursts of verbal aggression towards her that are completely out of character. He is less affectionate towards her and colder with people generally. He has become involved in rows with his neighbours, which never happened before. He has also been making inappropriate and lewd jokes and using made-up words, sometimes in public. He does not think that there is anything wrong with him. His MMSE score is 25. What is the most likely cause of his altered behaviour?

(a)   Lewy body dementia
(b)   Alzheimer's disease
(c)   Vascular dementia
(d)   **Frontotemporal dementia**
(e)   Depression

Frontotemporal dementia is the second-most common cause of dementia in people ≤65 years of age, with the highest incidence between 50 and 60 years of age. The core diagnostic features of frontotemporal dementia are insidious onset and gradual progression, early decline in regulation of social interpersonal conduct, early emotional blunting, and early loss of insight. Difficulties with language and speech are common, including perseveration, stereotypy and neologisms. Semantic problems (understanding the meaning and identity of words and objects) are disproportionately impaired, whereas episodic (autobiographical) memory is relatively well preserved (see further reading for current theories on this issue). Prognosis is poor and existing treatments focus on symptom control rather than slowing cognitive decline.

Although the term 'Pick's disease' was once used to represent a class of clinical syndromes with symptoms attributable to frontal and temporal lobe dysfunction, it is now used to mean a frontotemporal lobar degeneration due to specific pathological changes (Pick's bodies and Pick's cells). See Pasquier *et al* (2008) and, for further reading, Hornberger & Piguet (2012) and Nardell & Tampi (2014).

7   A 34-year-old man is referred to your out-patient clinic. He complains of low mood over the past 6 months. He also describes occasional difficulty in reading and writing and dressing himself. On full examination, he has difficulty in naming parts of objects, such as the second hand on your watch. Recently, he has been getting headaches. Where is the probable pathology?

    (a)   Cerebellum
    (b)   **Parietal lobe**
    (c)   Temporal lobe
    (d)   Frontal lobe
    (e)   Corpus callosum

This man is likely to have a parietal lobe lesion and will require further investigation, including brain imaging. Lesions in the parietal lobe are associated with impairment of core higher cognitive functions, including acalculia (inability to calculate), agraphia (inability to write), alexia (inability to read) and apraxia (inability to carry out learned skilled movements despite the retention of sensory and motor function). Other signs are subtle and require detailed and skilful clinical examination. These include astereognosis (inability to identify the shape and nature of an object by touch alone), agraphaesthesia (inability to identify a number traced on the hand) and finger agnosia (inability to recognise and name fingers despite the retention of sensation).

Parietal lobe lesions, including tumours, are less likely than frontal or temporal lobe pathology to present with psychological or behavioural changes; motor and sensory deficits are more common. Nonetheless, depression is not uncommon. See Talley & O'Connor (2010) and, for further reading, David *et al* (2009).

8   A 72-year-old woman is assessed at your clinic. Her husband is worried about her as she has 'not been herself' and has lost interest in things. She is not sleeping and has lost weight. She has been having a lot of physical health problems, including leg pain and abdominal cramps, and she is convinced she has cancer, although her GP has found nothing wrong. She denies feeling sad or upset. On cognitive assessment, she scores poorly, but this is mainly because she answers 'don't know' to most questions, even straightforward ones. What do you think her diagnosis is?

   (a)   Dementia
   (b)   Psychosis
   (c)   **Depression**
   (d)   Delirium
   (e)   No diagnosis

Depression in old age tends to present in a different way than at a younger age. The patient commonly focuses on physical symptoms and commonly minimises or has an under-expression of feelings of sadness. Somatic complaints might stem from depression rather than a physical cause. Psychotic symptoms are more common, although in this case the woman's beliefs about cancer are more likely to represent hypochondriasis, which is also common.

On cognitive examination, patients often perform poorly, but with a preponderance of 'don't know' answers, which suggests amotivation rather than cognitive impairment. This clinical observation led to the development of the term pseudodementia to describe poor cognitive performance due to depression, although the validity of this term has been called into question in recent years. Nonetheless, it is important to be aware of depression masquerading as dementia and/or physical illness in older adults. See Baldwin (2008) and Parmelee & Katz (1990) and, for further reading, Snowdon (2011).

9   A 78-year-old man with severe depressive illness is referred to your clinic and you start him on an antidepressant. A few weeks later, his GP writes to you informing you that he is stopping the antidepressant as it has resulted in hyponatraemia. What medication most likely to be the offending agent?

   (a)   Amitriptyline
   (b)   **Citalopram**
   (c)   Mirtazapine
   (d)   Duloxetine
   (e)   Trazadone

Pharmacological treatment of depression in the elderly can be difficult. The frequency and intensity of antidepressant-related adverse events is complicated by increased physical health problems and changes in physiology in older patients. There is no clear-cut guidance on the best antidepressant to use in a given situation and selection must be based on careful consideration of numerous factors, including the patient's physical condition and the side-effect profile of the medication.

SSRIs such as citalopram are non-sedative and are relatively free of interactions with other drugs. However, they can cause a range of side-effects, including gastrointestinal problems and hyponatraemia, particularly in the elderly. Use of higher doses of citalopram should be monitored with electrocardiograms because of increased risk of QTc prolongation. Mirtazapine is often used where insomnia is a problem, as it has a sedative effect at lower doses, whereas tricyclic antidepressants such as amitriptyline are used with caution because of risk of adverse cardiovascular events and withdrawal symptoms. See Baldwin (2008) and, for further reading, Jacob & Spinler (2006) and Wilkinson & Izmeth (2012).

10 A 23-year-old is assessed in the emergency department. He complains of a feeling of intense fear, associated with an odd sensation of having been in the exact same situation before. He describes having experienced an intense smell of rotting vegetables. All these sensations passed after a period of 1–2 min but for a time after he felt strange and then exhausted. The treating consultant suggests he might have had a seizure. Which type of seizure is he most likely to have had?

    (a)   Tonic–clonic seizure
    (b)   Absence seizure
    (c)   Atonic seizure
    (d)   **Temporal lobe epilepsy seizure**
    (e)   Non-epileptiform seizure

Temporal lobe epilepsy is a form of epilepsy where the origin of the seizure is the temporal lobe. It is the most common of the anatomically defined syndromes. Seizures can present with a wide range of symptoms, many of which mimic acute psychotic states. Compared with extratemporal seizures, episodes are typically of more gradual onset, usually feature a motionless stare and are relatively prolonged, lasting up to 2 min or occasionally even longer.

The feeling of fear this man experiences is called ictal fear and is a common type of aura, occurring in up to a quarter of temporal lobe epilepsy seizures. He is also experiencing déjà vu, which is another common feature. He describes olfactory hallucination, a symptom that should always arouse suspicion of organic pathology. Slow gradual recovery over several minutes and headaches are common. See Mellers (2009) and, for further reading, Thom & Bertram (2011).

11 Which two types of psychiatric disorder are most common in patients with epilepsy?

(a) **Depression and anxiety**
(b) Depression and psychosis
(c) Psychosis and anxiety
(d) OCD and depression
(e) OCD and psychosis

Psychiatric disorders can be divided into conditions associated with the cause of the epilepsy (e.g. intellectual disability, associated syndromes), disorders related to the seizures (e.g. pre-ictal states, intra-ictal symptoms, post-ictal delirium, psychosis) and conditions occurring between seizures thought to be associated with the condition (inter-ictal disorders).

Depression and anxiety are the most common of this last group, although estimates of incidence vary significantly. Symptoms of depression and anxiety can fall short of diagnostic criteria for full disorders, but still have significant morbidity. Rates are higher where there are ongoing seizures. The risk of suicide in epilepsy is high, with estimates of up to a 25-fold increase in risk, although other studies give more conservative estimates. Comorbid psychiatric illness is a major confounding factor for suicide risk and so diagnosis of this is crucial in patients with epilepsy. See Agrawal & Govender (2011), Christensen *et al* (2007) and Mellers (2009).

12 A 71-year-old woman with pneumonia becomes increasingly agitated throughout the course of an evening. She does not have a diagnosis of dementia but, during assessment, it is difficult to maintain her attention and she cannot tell you what day or date it is or where she is. She seems distracted and describes seeing insects climbing on the wall, although there are none there. What is this woman's probable diagnosis?

(a) Schizophrenia
(b) Depression
(c) New-onset Alzheimer's disease
(d) Parkinson's disease
(e) **Delirium**

This woman has delirium, which has most probably developed secondary to her pneumonia. Delirium is commonly referred to as an acute confusional state, although in recent times the concept of acute brain failure has emerged in the literature, along with recognition of more sub-acute and chronic forms of delirium. Treatment is a challenge, as there might be no clear-cut underlying cause and medications are contributing factors in a significant proportion of cases. Most pharmacological strategies are based on the theory of relative dopaminergic excess and cholinergic deficiency as the principal underlying neurochemical problem. Non-pharmacological interventions are also very important. See Hogg (2008) and, for further reading, Meagher & Leonard (2008).

13 A 36-year-old man is involved in a road traffic accident. He smashes his head against the window and is rendered unconscious. He loses consciousness for several minutes but then begins to recover. He is taken to hospital to be assessed. Which type of memory loss is most common in such injuries?

(a) Retrograde memory loss
(b) Procedural memory loss
(c) **Anterograde memory loss**
(d) Semantic memory loss
(e) Working memory loss

Anterograde memory loss after head injury, or post-traumatic amnesia, is defined as an amnesic gap from the moment of injury to the resumption of normal continuous memory. The recovery is usually gradual, from unconsciousness, through a period of being conscious and alert but amnesic, to full recovery of day-to-day memory. Even in milder injuries, where there is no significant post-traumatic loss of consciousness, there might be a time period in which events fail to be recorded in memory and there is an amnesic gap.

Evidence suggests that episodic memory is typically more impaired than procedural memory during this period and patients can learn new skills during this time while not remembering day-to-day events. Retrograde amnesia is relatively less common and, except in rare cases, much shorter than post-traumatic amnesia. See Fleminger (2009).

14 A 17-year-old boy is brought to hospital after collapsing on the rugby field following a collision. Which investigation will be most useful in assessing injury to his brain?

(a) Skull X-ray
(b) Magnetic resonance imaging (MRI) spectroscopy of the brain
(c) Electroencephalogram
(d) Positron emission tomography (PET)
(e) **Computed tomography (CT) of the brain**

Although all the investigations here might be considered, computed tomography (CT) of the brain is the best choice in this situation. CT is an effective, practical and easy-to-use investigative tool for head injuries. Non-contrast CT is the modality of choice in the first 24 h after a head injury, as it is effective at identifying extra-axial and intra-axial haemorrhages, as well as bony injuries.

Magnetic resonance imaging (MRI) spectroscopy may also be considered, as it is superior at identifying injuries at the brain–bone interface and at identifying white-matter changes caused by diffuse axonal injury due to brain trauma. Positron emission tomography (PET) provides functional rather than anatomical information and is mainly a research tool at present.

Head injuries in sport have become an increasing cause for concern in recent times, particularly in high-impact sports such as rugby. See Fleminger (2009) and, for further reading, Kim & Gean (2011) and McKee *et al* (2009).

15 A 37-year-old woman presents reporting feeling anxious, hyperactive and irritable most of the time for the past 2 months. She also complains of weight loss (despite an increased appetite), intolerance to heat, hair loss, muscle aches, weakness, fatigue and intermittent diarrhoea. Which of the following endocrine conditions is most likely to explain her symptoms?

(a) Diabetes mellitus
(b) Addison's disease
(c) Phaeochromocytoma
(d) Diabetes insipidus
(e) **Hyperthyroidism**

Assessment of thyroid function is important in psychiatry. Thyroid abnormalities are common in the general population and thyroid function tests should be carried our routinely as part of an organic work-up. Psychological disturbance of some degree is universal with hyperthyroidism, which results in autonomic overarousal. Patients frequently complain of nervousness and fatigue, and seem restless, overactive and irritable, sometimes with hyperacuity of perception and over-reaction to noise. Generalised anxiety has been reported in up to 80% and depression can be prominent, with symptoms of agitation rather than psychomotor retardation. Hyperthyroidism also accounts for this woman's other physical symptoms.

Phaeochromocytomas can lead to pronounced anxiety and irritability due to sympathetic hyperactivity. However, this tends to occur in episodes that last less than 1 h and does not explain the range of physical symptoms here. See Harrison & Kopelman (2009) and, for further reading, Brandt *et al* (2014).

16 A 68-year-old man is referred to your clinic. He holds the fixed belief that his neighbours are entering his house by passing through the walls. He says he can hear their voices in his living room even when he cannot see them there. He does not have first-rank symptoms of schizophrenia. He does not have low or elevated mood. He scores 30/30 on the MMSE, is orientated to time, place and person and does not have visual hallucinations. What is his most likely diagnosis?

(a) Alzheimer's disease
(b) Depression
(c) Mania
(d) **Late-onset schizophrenia**
(e) Delirium

Although relatively uncommon, schizophrenia can occur later in life as an independent cause of delusional beliefs and other psychotic symptoms. Recent evidence suggests that late-onset schizophrenia is a subtype of schizophrenia that is more common in women, has less severe positive symptoms and general psychopathology, and has less severe impairment in abstraction/cognitive flexibility, verbal memory and everyday functioning.

This man is describing a partition delusion, which is found in two-thirds of cases. When assessing perceptual abnormalities in older people, it is essential to rule out other causes of altered perception, such as impending deafness or blindness, which can lead to hallucinations or hallucinatory-type experiences. He does not have other features suggestive of dementia, delirium or affective illness, although a thorough screening should always be carried out, as these diagnoses are more common. See Howard (2008) and, for further reading, Vahia *et al* (2010).

EMI answers

Cognitive assessment

Options:

- (a) MMSE
- (b) Addenbrooke's Cognitive Examination
- (c) Frontal lobe battery
- (d) Astereognosis and agraphesthesia
- (e) Spelling WORLD backwards
- (f) Registration and recall
- (g) Difficulty naming dates of World War II
- (h) Intersecting pentagons

Match the items above with the items below. (Each option is used once only.)

1 A screening and monitoring test for cognitive impairment
   (a) MMSE

2 A test of visuospatial skills
   (h) Intersecting pentagons

3 Tested using 'apple, penny, table' in MMSE
   (f) Registration and recall

4 Indicates semantic memory impairment
   (g) Difficulty naming dates of World War II

5 Indicates parietal lobe impairment
   (d) Astereognosis and agraphesthesia

6 Tests language skills in more detail than MMSE
   (b) Addenbrooke's Cognitive Examination

7 Includes Luria test and 'go/no-go' test
   (c) Frontal lobe battery

8 Test of attention
   (e) Spelling WORLD backwards

Medications in old age psychiatry

Options:

- (a) Donepezil
- (b) Mirtazapine
- (c) Second-generation antipsychotics
- (d) Haloperidol
- (e) Galantamine
- (f) SNRIs
- (g) SSRIs

Match the items above with the answers below. (More than one answer may be given for each item below.)

1 Acetylcholinesterase inhibitors used in dementia

(a) Donepezil

(e) Galantamine

2 Particular caution advised in the elderly because of risk of cerebrovascular adverse events

(c) Second-generation antipsychotics

3 First-line antidepressants used in the elderly

(f) SNRIs

(g) SSRIs

4 Another antidepressant used in the elderly

(b) Mirtazapine

Symptoms, signs and test results

Options:

- (a) Jerky, random and uncontrollable movements in a 40-year-old man
- (b) Visual hallucination
- (c) Fluctuating cognitive impairment
- (d) Genetic test indicating autosomal dominant condition
- (e) Hyperthermia and muscle rigidity
- (f) Highly impaired attention on mental state exam
- (g) Resting tremor and bradykinesia
- (h) Agitation that is worse at night
- (i) Highly elevated creatine phosphokinase

Match the items above with the answers below. (Each answer below has more than one matching item. Each item may be used more than once.)

1 Lewy body dementia

(b) Visual hallucination

(c) Fluctuating cognitive impairment

(g) Resting tremor and bradykinesia

2 Huntington's disease
   (a) Jerky, random and uncontrollable movements in a 40-year-old man
   (d) Genetic test indicating autosomal dominant condition

3 Neuroleptic malignant syndrome
   (e) Hyperthermia and muscle rigidity
   (i) Highly elevated creatine phosphokinase

4 Delirium
   (b) Visual hallucination
   (c) Fluctuating cognitive impairment
   (f) Highly impaired attention on mental state exam
   (h) Agitation that is worse at night

CHAPTER 6

Child and adolescent psychiatry

MCQs

1 The parents of a 4-year-old boy have returned to your clinic for a follow-up appointment. Their son was recently diagnosed with autism spectrum disorder. All the following are characteristic of a diagnosis of autism spectrum disorder, except:

   (a) Stereotyped or repetitive motor movements, use of objects, or speech
   (b) Highly restricted, fixated interests that are abnormal in intensity or focus
   (c) Exceptionally gifted in a specific domain (e.g. memory, music)
   (d) Deficits in non-verbal communicative behaviours used for social interaction
   (e) Deficits in developing, maintaining, and understanding relationships

2 A couple attends the clinic, concerned that their 4-year-old son has yet to speak. Following a comprehensive clinical assessment, you consider a diagnosis of autism spectrum disorder. All the following would be appropriate investigations in this assessment except for:

   (a) Use of screening and diagnostic instruments
   (b) Genetic testing
   (c) IQ assessment
   (d) Speech and language assessment
   (e) Magnetic resonance imaging of the brain

3 After receiving a diagnosis of autism spectrum disorder, an adolescent boy, prompted by his parents, seeks information from you about his condition. Which of the following is true?

   (a) Autism spectrum disorder is more common in females
   (b) There is little genetic risk
   (c) Prevalence has decreased over the past decade
   (d) Use of the measles, mumps and rubella (MMR) vaccine is associated with an increased risk of autism
   (e) The risk of any future siblings having the condition is approximately 1 in 10

4   A 12-year-old girl presents to the clinic with a 3-month history of educational and social decline. On examination, she reports third-person auditory hallucinations, delusions of reference and somatic passivity. All the following regarding a diagnosis of early-onset schizophrenia are incorrect, except:

(a)   Incidence of psychosis by 13 years of age is approximately 1 in 10 000

ϯ (b)   The earlier onset has a better prognosis than adult-onset psychosis

(c)   Rapid titration of antipsychotic treatment is indicated in adolescents with first-episode psychosis

(d)   Clozapine should not be considered for use in children

(e)   Evidence of psychotic symptoms excludes a differential diagnosis of epilepsy

5   A 14-year-old girl attends the out-patient clinic. She is having a moderate depressive episode of 6 months' duration with an associated decline in educational performance. There is no associated suicidal ideation or plan. Which of the following would be the most appropriate first-line treatment intervention?

(a)   An elective admission to the regional child and adolescent in-patient unit to commence treatment

(b)   Fluoxetine

(c)   Watchful waiting

(d)   Cognitive–behavioural therapy

(e)   Diet and exercise advice

6   A 16-year-old boy attends the clinic with a recurrence of depressive illness. He had previously responded well to a combination of fluoxetine and cognitive–behavioural therapy and was discharged to GP follow-up 3 months ago. All the following would indicate a need for hospitalisation, except?

(a)   Poor sleep

(b)   Suicidal ideation

(c)   Prior suicide attempt when depressed

(d)   Command hallucinations

(e)   Lack of family support

7   A 7-year-old boy attends the assessment clinic accompanied by his parents. He was referred by his GP for an assessment for ADHD, after his teacher raised concerns with his parents about his poor attention in class. All the following are core features of ADHD except:

(a)   Impulsivity

(b)   Distractibility

(c)   Inability to sustain focus

(d)   Fidgeting

(e)   Restricted pattern of interests

8   A 6-year-old girl is referred to your out-patient clinic after concerns expressed by her teacher that she is falling behind in class because of constant daydreaming. The following are symptoms of inattention in ADHD, except:

(a)   Doesn't seem to listen
(b)   Forgetfulness
(c)   Poor organisation
(d)   Difficulty in engaging in tasks quietly
(e)   Avoids tasks requiring sustained mental effort

9   You assess a 7-year-old girl at the clinic who was referred for an assessment of hyperactivity. All the following are symptoms of hyperactivity–impulsivity in ADHD, except:

(a)   Distractibility
(b)   Excessive talking
(c)   Interrupting
(d)   Difficulty in waiting for their turn
(e)   Blurting out answers

10 At the weekly ADHD clinic, your consultant asks you to carefully assess the attending adolescents for comorbid conditions. All the following are conditions associated with ADHD, except:

(a)   PTSD
(b)   Bipolar affective disorder
(c)   OCD
(d)   Substance misuse disorders
(e)   Depression

11 An 8-year-old boy attending the clinic has been diagnosed with ADHD. The appropriate first-line treatment is:

(a)   Atomoxetine
(b)   Diazepam
(c)   Methylphenidate
(d)   Behaviour management techniques
(e)   Dexamfetamine

12 A 10-year-old boy with a diagnosis of ADHD has been treated with methylphenidate for the past 3 years. His mother is concerned that he might be developing adverse effects due to the treatment. Which of the following is a common adverse effect associated with the use of methylphenidate?

(a)   Growth restriction
(b)   Bradycardia
(c)   Weight gain
(d)   Sedation
(e)   Early morning wakening

EMI questions

Diagnosis

Options:

- (a) ADHD
- (b) Depression
- (c) Intellectual disability
- (d) Oppositional defiant disorder
- (e) Early-onset schizophrenia
- (f) Autism spectrum disorder
- (g) Separation anxiety
- (h) Elective mutism

For each of the following clinical vignettes, please select the probable diagnosis:

1   A 4-year-old boy has a history of poor social interaction and delayed language development, and engages in a pattern of restricted and often repetitive behaviours. All these were evident before the age of 3.

2   A 13-year-old boy has recently started to refuse to attend school. He has also become more isolated from his family and friends, is sleeping poorly and has lost weight because of a declining appetite.

3   The teacher of an 8-year-old boy describes a pattern of angry moods, argumentative, disobedient and disruptive behaviour, and vindictiveness towards classmates over the last 6 months.

Diagnosis

Options:

- (a) Attention deficit hyperactivity disorder
- (b) Autism spectrum disorder
- (c) Intellectual disability
- (d) Elective mutism
- (e) Conduct disorder
- (f) Enuresis
- (g) Encopresis
- (h) Tic disorder

For each of the following clinical vignettes, please select the probable diagnosis:

1   A 14-year-old boy is referred to your clinic after being expelled from school for persistent aggressive and bullying behaviour. He was recently arrested for stealing from shops and has previously burgled houses. He uses alcohol and cannabis with friends.

2 A 5-year-old girl is referred to the clinic by her GP. She has been having frequent episodes of bed-wetting and has started wetting herself during the day. She was previously toilet trained and this is a recent-onset problem that started after the birth of her brother 6 months ago.

3 A 12-year-old boy is referred to the clinic for an assessment of ADHD. On assessment, you find that he has frequent twitching movements of his eyelids and shoulder shrugging, which have been recurrent on a daily basis for more than a year.

MCQ answers

1 The parents of a 4-year-old boy have returned to your clinic for a follow-up appointment. Their son was recently diagnosed with autism spectrum disorder. All the following are characteristic of a diagnosis of autism spectrum disorder, except:

(a) Stereotyped or repetitive motor movements, use of objects, or speech
(b) Highly restricted, fixated interests that are abnormal in intensity or focus
(c) **Exceptionally gifted in a specific domain (e.g. memory, music)**
(d) Deficits in non-verbal communicative behaviours used for social interaction
(e) Deficits in developing, maintaining, and understanding relationships

The core features of autism spectrum disorder in DSM-5 are restricted, repetitive patterns of behaviour, interests, or activities and persistent deficits in social communication and social interaction across multiple contexts. In DSM-IV, language delay was a defining feature of autism (autistic disorder), but it is not included in DSM-5. Approximately 45% of individuals with ASD have an intellectual disability (although for the DSM-IV diagnosis of autism, a 75% prevalence of intellectual disability was reported). Although a minority of patients with autism spectrum disorder might have well-developed skills in a specific functional domain, this is not the case for most and is not a characteristic feature of the disorder. See APA (2013).

2 A couple attends the clinic, concerned that their 4-year-old son has yet to speak. Following a comprehensive clinical assessment, you consider a diagnosis of autism spectrum disorder. All the following would be appropriate investigations in this assessment except for:

(a) Use of screening and diagnostic instruments
(b) Genetic testing
(c) IQ assessment
(d) Speech and language assessment
(e) **Magnetic resonance imaging of the brain**

A multidisciplinary approach to investigation should be instigated, including a speech and language assessment (to exclude disorders that affect speech and language) and an IQ assessment. There are no standard blood investigations recommended for the assessment of autism spectrum disorder and no biomarkers have been identified. A laboratory work-up might include genetic testing for conditions like fragile X syndrome if the child had any of the following features: diagnosed or possible intellectual disability, family history of intellectual disability, or dysmorphic facial features. Fragile X syndrome has high comorbidity with autism spectrum disorder. Screening and diagnostic instruments, such as the autism diagnostic observation schedule and the diagnostic interview for social and communication disorders, are used by the multidisciplinary team to aid in diagnosis. There is currently no clinical evidence to support the role of routine clinical neuroimaging in the diagnostic evaluation of autism. See Lai *et al* (2014).

3   After receiving a diagnosis of autism spectrum disorder, an adolescent boy, prompted
     by his parents, seeks information from you about his condition. Which of the
     following is true?
     (a)   Autism spectrum disorder is more common in females
     (b)   There is little genetic risk
     (c)   Prevalence has decreased over the past decade
     (d)   Use of the measles, mumps and rubella (MMR) vaccine is associated with an
            increased risk of autism
     (e)   **The risk of any future siblings having the condition is approximately
            1 in 10**

Autism spectrum disorder has a population prevalence of at least 0.6%, with evidence that the prevalence has increased over the past two decades, particularly for individuals without intellectual disability. Approximately 50% of those with autism spectrum disorder are of normal learning ability. It occurs more frequently in men, with a male:female ratio of 3:1 (approximately 10:1 for DSM-IV diagnosed autism with speech delays/language impairment). Twin studies have suggested that autism has high heritability (> 80%), indicating that genetic risk is a major factor in its development. The recurrence risk of autism spectrum disorders (i.e. the rate of recurrence in a younger sibling) is estimated to be between 3% and 10% (although a longitudinal study indicates that the risk might be higher, at 19%). For more narrowly defined autism, the recurrence rate in siblings is 3%.

A small case series from 1998 linked the onset of autism to the measles, mumps and rubella (MMR) vaccine, sparking a vaccine scare and a reduction in the rates of MMR vaccination in the UK, with measles becoming endemic by 2008. This paper was deeply flawed, both ethically and scientifically. It was retracted in 2010 and its author discredited and struck off the UK medical register. Subsequent epidemiological studies have consistently found no evidence of a link between the MMR vaccine and autism. See Godlee *et al* (2011), Lai *et al* (2014) and Ozonoff *et al* (2011).

4 A 12-year-old girl presents to the clinic with a 3-month history of educational and social decline. On examination, she reports third-person auditory hallucinations, delusions of reference and somatic passivity. All the following regarding a diagnosis of early-onset schizophrenia are false, except:

(a) **Incidence of psychosis by 13 years of age is approximately 1 in 10000**
(b) The earlier onset has a better prognosis than adult-onset psychosis
(c) Rapid titration of antipsychotic treatment is indicated in adolescents with first-episode psychosis
(d) Clozapine should not be considered for use in children
(e) Evidence of psychotic symptoms excludes a differential diagnosis of epilepsy

Early-onset schizophrenia is extremely rare, with an incidence rate of 1 in 10000. Earlier age at onset of a psychotic illness is associated with a worse prognosis. Antipsychotic medications should be used in combination with psychological therapies and family support. They should be prescribed at a low dose initially and gradually titrated with close monitoring for evidence of adverse effects and toxicity.

Clozapine can be used in children and adolescents. In the Treatment of Early-Onset Schizophrenia Spectrum Disorders (TEOSS) study, although treatment resulted in symptomatic improvement, the response rates were below 50% for all first-line antipsychotic medications examined. The poor response highlights the clinical severity of early-onset schizophrenia, which is associated with greater disease burden and psychosocial disability. Despite this evidence for efficacy of clozapine in this age group, in both the short and longer term, its use in paediatric patients is very restricted. The most significant obstacle is the limited information regarding its adverse effects. See Gogtay & Rapoport (2008) and Sikich et al (2008).

5 A 14-year-old girl attends the out-patient clinic. She is having a moderate depressive episode of 6 months' duration with an associated decline in educational performance. There is no associated suicidal ideation or plan. Which of the following would be the most appropriate first-line treatment intervention?

(a) An elective admission to the regional child and adolescent in-patient unit to commence treatment
(b) Fluoxetine
(c) Watchful waiting
(d) **Cognitive–behavioural therapy**
(e) Diet and exercise advice

Treatment for a moderate depressive episode should be initiated and a watchful-waiting approach is not appropriate. Cognitive–behavioural therapy is the first-line treatment option and has been shown to be effective in the treatment of mild and moderate depressive episodes in children and adolescents. Evidence from randomised clinical trials suggests efficacy in the treatment of moderate to severe depressive episodes using one of three SSRIs: fluoxetine, sertraline, and citalopram. Fluoxetine is the only one of these licensed in the UK for the treatment of depression in adolescents.

In 2003, it was thought SSRIs might be associated with an increased suicide risk in young people. Epidemiological work indicates that this warning led to reductions in antidepressant use and a possible increase in suicide in young people. Antidepressants should be prescribed for young people when indicated, but patients should be closely monitored in the early stages of treatment for emerging anxiety, agitation or suicidal ideation.

If the patient had developed psychotic symptoms secondary to depression or was suicidal and had poor family support, then a hospital admission could be considered. See Taylor *et al* (2012).

6   A 16-year-old boy attends the clinic with a recurrence of depressive illness. He had previously responded well to a combination of fluoxetine and cognitive–behavioural therapy and was discharged to GP follow-up 3 months ago. All the following would indicate a need for hospitalisation, except?

   (a)   **Poor sleep**
   (b)   Suicidal ideation
   (c)   Prior suicide attempt when depressed
   (d)   Command hallucinations
   (e)   Lack of family support

Poor sleep is not an indication for hospital admission and could be managed in the community. All the other factors are risk factors for suicide in an adolescent who is depressed and suggest a need for in-patient treatment. See Pelkonen & Marttunen (2003).

7   A 7-year-old boy attends the assessment clinic accompanied by his parents. He was referred by his GP for an assessment for ADHD, after his teacher raised concerns with his parents about his poor attention in class. All the following are core features of ADHD except:

   (a)   Impulsivity
   (b)   Distractibility
   (c)   Inability to sustain focus
   (d)   Fidgeting
   (e)   **Restricted pattern of interests**

ADHD is the most frequently occurring neurobiological disorder in childhood and is characterised by inattention, impulsivity and hyperactivity that are excessive when compared with other individuals at the same developmental level and that have an onset before 12 years of age (DSM-5; < 7 years of age in the ICD-10 diagnostic criteria). The symptoms should be present for more than 6 months, in multiple settings (for example, home and school or a healthcare setting), and cause functional impairment for the child.

The worldwide prevalence of ADHD is estimated to be 5.9–7.1% in children and adolescents and 5.0% in adults (based on DSM-IV criteria). On the basis of the narrower criteria of ICD-10, hyperkinetic disorder (equivalent to severe ADHD and describing the occurrence of all three hyperactivity, impulsivity and inattention symptoms) is estimated to occur in about 1–2% of children and young people in the UK. There is a male preponderance, with a male:female ratio of 3:1. See Feldman & Reiff (2014) and Hill (2015).

8   A 6-year-old girl is referred to your out-patient clinic after concerns expressed by her teacher that she is falling behind in class because of constant daydreaming. The following are symptoms of inattention in ADHD, except:

(a)   Doesn't seem to listen
(b)   Forgetfulness
(c)   Poor organisation
(d)   **Difficulty in engaging in tasks quietly**
(e)   Avoids tasks requiring sustained mental effort

The main symptoms of ADHD include inattention (e.g. failing to pay close attention to details; difficulty sustaining attention and with organisation; distractibility; forgetfulness), hyperactivity and impulsivity (e.g. fidgeting; difficulty remaining seated; running about excessively; excessive talking and interrupting; blurting out answers; difficulty in waiting for their turn).

DSM-5 divides ADHD into three subtypes: predominantly inattentive, predominantly hyperactive–impulsive, and combined presentations. The predominantly inattentive and predominantly hyperactive–impulsive presentations both require six of nine symptoms in children and five of nine symptoms in adolescents and adults (≥ 17 years). The combined presentation requires that the criteria for both inattentive and hyperactive–impulsive presentations are met. Symptoms must be present for at least 6 months, and the behaviours must be present and create significant difficulties for the person in at least two different settings (e.g. home and school). See APA (2013) and Hill (2015).

9   You assess a 7-year-old girl at the clinic who was referred for an assessment of hyper-activity. All the following are symptoms of hyperactivity–impulsivity in ADHD, except:

(a)   **Distractibility**
(b)   Excessive talking
(c)   Interrupting
(d)   Difficulty in waiting for their turn
(e)   Blurting out answers

Distractibility is a symptom of inattention in ADHD (see answer to question 8). See APA (2013) and Hill (2015).

10   At the weekly ADHD clinic, your consultant asks you to carefully assess the attending adolescents for comorbid conditions. All the following are conditions associated with ADHD, except:

(a)   **PTSD**
(b)   Bipolar affective disorder
(c)   OCD
(d)   Substance misuse disorders
(e)   Depression

The symptoms of ADHD can overlap with the symptoms of other related disorders, and therefore care in making a diagnosis is needed. Common conditions coexisting with ADHD are: in children – disorders of mood, anxiety, conduct, learning, motor control and communication; in adolescents and adults – bipolar disorder, OCD and substance misuse.

In fact, there is mounting evidence that ADHD is an important (but up to now scarcely studied) risk factor in the development and persistence of substance misuse in adolescents and adults.

ADHD is associated with an early age at onset of substance misuse, a more rapid transition into more severe types of substance misuse, and a more problematic course of the substance use disorders, including more difficulty in reaching remission. Available studies (conducted mostly in the United States) suggest that ADHD is present in 10–25% of adults with substance misuse disorders. See Gleason & Castle (2012).

11 An 8-year-old boy attending the clinic has been diagnosed with ADHD. The appropriate first-line treatment is:
  (a) Atomoxetine
  (b) Diazepam
  (c) Methylphenidate
  (d) **Behaviour management techniques**
  (e) Dexamfetamine

The first-line intervention for a child with ADHD is non-pharmacological treatment. Psychosocial interventions consist of training parents in behavioural management, parent training and education programmes, consultation with teachers/school personnel and individual work (e.g. cognitive–behavioural therapy, social skills training) with the child. Parents can receive training in general operant conditioning techniques, such as contingent application of reinforcement or punishment in response to appropriate/inappropriate behaviours. Reinforcement procedures typically rely on praise, privileges or tokens, whereas punishment methods usually involve loss of positive attention, privileges or tokens, or formal 'time out' from reinforcement.

If there is no response to psychosocial interventions, or if the child presents with severe ADHD, then pharmacological treatment should be initiated. Determining the severity of the disorder should be a matter for clinical judgement, taking into account the severity of impairment, pervasiveness of symptoms, individual factors and familial and social context. Pharmacological approaches to treatment consist of the use of stimulant medication, such as methylphenidate (first line), and non-stimulants, such as atomoxetine (second line). Amphetamine-based salts are used for treatment-resistant ADHD. Combined pharmacological and non-pharmacological treatments are commonly used. See Antshel *et al* (2011).

12 A 10-year-old boy with a diagnosis of ADHD has been treated with methylphenidate for the past 3 years. His mother is concerned that he might be developing adverse effects due to the treatment. Which of the following is a common adverse effect associated with the use of methylphenidate?

(a) **Growth restriction**
(b) Bradycardia
(c) Weight gain
(d) Sedation
(e) Early morning wakening

The drug treatment of ADHD should be part of a comprehensive treatment programme. The choice of medication should take into consideration comorbid conditions (e.g. tics and cardiac problems) and assess for family history of heart disease or sudden cardiac death.

Methylphenidate is a central nervous system (CNS) stimulant. CNS stimulants are primarily prescribed for children with severe and persistent symptoms of ADHD. Children with moderate symptoms of ADHD can be treated with CNS stimulants when psychological interventions have been unsuccessful or are unavailable. Treatment often needs to be continued into adolescence, and might need to be continued into adulthood (65% of patients have symptoms persisting into adulthood and 25–30% meet the criteria for adult ADHD). The prescription of methylphenidate in children should be accompanied by regular monitoring of height and weight (to monitor for growth restriction) and heart rate and blood pressure (to monitor for repeated tachycardia and hypertension). See Joint Formulary Committee (2014) and NICE (2008).

EMI answers

Diagnosis

Options:

(a) ADHD
(b) Depression
(c) Intellectual disability
(d) Oppositional defiant disorder
(e) Early-onset schizophrenia
(f) Autism spectrum disorder
(g) Separation anxiety
(h) Elective mutism

For each of the following clinical vignettes, please select the probable diagnosis:

1 A 4-year-old boy has a history of poor social interaction and delayed language development, and engages in a pattern of restricted and often repetitive behaviours. All these were evident before the age of 3.

(f) Autism spectrum disorder

2   A 13-year-old boy has recently started to refuse to attend school. He has also become more isolated from his family and friends, is sleeping poorly and has lost weight because of a declining appetite.

(b) Depression

3   The teacher of an 8-year-old boy describes a pattern of angry moods, argumentative, disobedient and disruptive behaviour, and vindictiveness towards classmates over the last 6 months.

(d) Oppositional defiant disorder

Diagnosis

Options:

- (a)   Attention deficit hyperactivity disorder
- (b)   Autism spectrum disorder
- (c)   Intellectual disability
- (d)   Elective mutism
- (e)   Conduct disorder
- (f)   Enuresis
- (g)   Encopresis
- (h)   Tic disorder

For each of the following clinical vignettes, please select the probable diagnosis:

1   A 14-year-old boy is referred to your clinic after being expelled from school for persistent aggressive and bullying behaviour. He was recently arrested for stealing from shops and has previously burgled houses. He uses alcohol and cannabis with friends.

(e) Conduct disorder

2   A 5-year-old girl is referred to the clinic by her GP. She has been having frequent episodes of bed-wetting and has started wetting herself during the day. She was previously toilet trained and this is a recent-onset problem that started after the birth of her brother 6 months ago.

(f) Enuresis

3   A 12-year-old boy is referred to the clinic for an assessment of ADHD. On assessment, he does not display inattention or hyperactivity, but you find he has frequent twitching movements of his eyelids and shoulder shrugging, which have been recurrent on a daily basis for more than a year.

(h) Tic disorder

CHAPTER 7

Disorders of personality, behaviour and eating

MCQs

1 Which of the following is not true of behaviours in personality disorder according to ICD-10?

 (a) An enduring pattern that deviates markedly from the culturally expected range
 (b) Occurs across a broad range of personal and social situations
 (c) Causes personal distress
 (d) Onset is in early adulthood
 (e) Is inflexible, maladaptive, or otherwise dysfunctional

2 An 18-year-old woman presents to the emergency department with superficial, self-inflicted cuts to her arms. She said that she did this to relieve tension, as she has been feeling very low in mood and does not have hope for the future. However, her mother says that earlier in the day she seemed to be in a good mood and was laughing with her in the kitchen. When they later argued, she became very angry and began to scream at her mother, saying that no one loved her. She has a very unstable relationship with her boyfriend and she is preoccupied with her weight and uncertain about her sexuality. What is the most likely diagnosis here?

 (a) Depression
 (b) Bipolar disorder
 (c) Emotionally unstable personality disorder
 (d) Anorexia nervosa
 (e) Schizoid personality disorder

3 Anankastic personality disorder shares some characteristics with which other psychiatric disorder?
   (a) Generalised anxiety disorder
   (b) Panic disorder
   (c) PTSD
   (d) Agoraphobia
   (e) OCD

4 A 34-year-old man is referred to the out-patient clinic, reporting ongoing difficulties with his landlord. He has been in several arguments with him and says that his landlord is to blame for these. He admits that he drinks late into the night, but denies his landlord's accusations that he is playing loud music and shouting. He has several arrests for assaults and has been violent to previous girlfriends, with whom he has only had short-term relationships. He does not understand why his last girlfriend was upset when he hit her. What type of personality disorder does this man have?
   (a) Schizoid
   (b) Dissocial/antisocial
   (c) Schizotypal
   (d) Emotionally unstable
   (e) Narcissistic

5 A 22-year-old university student is referred by his GP as she is concerned that he might be psychotic. He spends hours each day playing computer games and watching fantasy epic films and programmes. He speaks a lot about characters from these programmes and how he relates to them. He does not have any close friends or intimate relationships. He dresses in a strange, dishevelled manner and is not responsive to concerns expressed by peers and lecturers about his personal hygiene. His mother says that he was an odd, withdrawn child who showed little affection for his siblings and that his behaviour has not changed in recent years. On assessment, the psychiatrist feels that he has a personality disorder, rather than psychosis. What disorder does he diagnose?
   (a) Antisocial
   (b) Schizoid
   (c) Schizotypal
   (d) Emotionally unstable
   (e) Narcissistic

6   Which of the following is not a core feature of schizotypal disorder?
    (a)   Inappropriate or constricted affect
    (b)   Behaviour or appearance that is odd, eccentric, or peculiar
    (c)   Poor rapport with others and a tendency to social withdrawal
    (d)   Inability to maintain enduring relationships, although no difficulty
          in establishing them
    (e)   Occasional quasi-psychotic episodes with illusions, hallucinations
          and delusion-like ideas

7   A 20-year-old student is referred to your clinic because of her GP's
    concerns about her weight loss. She has lost several kilograms in recent
    weeks and her BMI is now 16.5. She is continuing to attend university
    and sees no problem with her weight. In fact she believes she should
    lose more as she is 'still a bit fat'. She has stopped having periods. Which
    of the following features are not supportive of a diagnosis of anorexia
    nervosa?
    (a)   Self-induced vomiting and purging
    (b)   Excessive exercise
    (c)   Use of appetite suppressants and diuretics
    (d)   Dark hair on arms and legs
    (e)   Preoccupation with food

8   A 45-year-old teacher is having difficulty at work. He believes his
    colleagues are plotting against him and that they wish to force him
    to leave his job. He has had confrontations with several colleagues
    in which he has cited human rights law, and has threatened to use a
    solicitor. When one colleague asked him about his weekend plans, he
    was convinced this meant she was suggesting that he clear out his desk.
    He believes that it is right that he be promoted to vice-principal as he
    is clearly the best teacher in the school. He has left or been asked to
    leave four previous schools because of similar problems. What is the
    likely diagnosis?
    (a)   Antisocial personality disorder
    (b)   Schizophrenia
    (c)   Delusional disorder
    (d)   Paranoid personality disorder
    (e)   Narcissistic personality disorder

9   An underweight 19-year-old woman with a BMI of 16 kg/m², and a history of self-induced vomiting, dietary restriction and a morbid fear of fatness presents to an out-patient clinic. Which of the following psychological treatments is not recommended in the NICE guidelines for treatment of her condition?

    (a)   Psychoanalysis
    (b)   Cognitive–behavioural therapy
    (c)   Interpersonal psychotherapy
    (d)   Cognitive analytic therapy
    (e)   Family interventions focused explicitly on eating disorders

10 A 25-year-old accountant attends your out-patient clinic, reporting low mood. When you explore her story, it becomes clear that food plays a very important role in her life. She speaks of craving food a lot of the time and describes binging on large amounts of cake and chocolates, often alone in her room. She admits that sometimes she induces vomiting. She is of normal weight but feels she is too fat. Which pharmacological treatment is indicated for her condition?

    (a)   Tricyclic antidepressant
    (b)   SSRI
    (c)   First-generation antipsychotic
    (d)   Second-generation antipsychotic
    (e)   Benzodiazepine

11 The mother of a 21-year-old woman attending your clinic asks to meet you. She is worried that her daughter has an eating disorder. She had some problems with binge-eating when she was younger. Which of the following is true about eating disorders?

    (a)   They are more common in males than females
    (b)   Genetic factors are not important
    (c)   Environmental factors are important
    (d)   They are more common in low-income countries
    (e)   They do not affect mortality

12 A 35-year-old businessman enjoys dressing up in his wife's clothes. He says he does so to experience what it feels like to be a woman and it does not cause him sexual arousal. He has no desire to be a woman. What is the correct term to describe his behaviour?

    (a)   Transsexualism
    (b)   Dual-role transvestism
    (c)   Fetishism
    (d)   Fetishistic transvestism
    (e)   Exhibitionism

13 A 34-year-old man is involved in a minor road accident. He has a small bruise on his neck but no pain or dysfunction. He tells his wife he is hoping to get a payout from his insurance company. He tells his GP he has severe back pain and PTSD and is referred to you for assessment. What is the correct term to describe his behaviour?

(a) Factitious disorder (Munchausen's syndrome)
(b) Malingering
(c) Conversion disorder
(d) Somatoform disorder
(e) Elaboration of physical symptoms for psychological reasons

14 A 56-year-old woman spends half of her weekly budget on gaming scratch cards. She makes small wins but ultimately loses financially each week. She has repeatedly tried to stop doing this but has failed. It causes her a lot of distress as she is not well off and it also interrupts her working and leisure routine. She has intrusive thoughts about buying scratch cards when she is at work. What is her diagnosis?

(a) Trichotillomania
(b) Pathological gambling
(c) No diagnosis
(d) Kleptomania
(e) Other habit and impulse disorder

EMI questions

Personality disorder traits

Options:

(a) Self-dramatisation
(b) Excessive preoccupation with being criticised or rejected in social situations
(c) Unwillingness to become involved with people unless certain of being liked
(d) Encouraging or allowing others to make most of one's own important life decisions
(e) Subordination of one's own needs to those of others on whom one is dependent
(f) Continual seeking for excitement and activities in which the patient is the centre of attention
(g) Inappropriate seductiveness in appearance or behaviour
(h) Restrictions in lifestyle because of need to have physical security

The items above are traits of which personality disorder? (There is more than one item for each answer.)

1 Histrionic personality disorder. (Select three options.)
2 Anxious/avoidant personality disorder. (Select three options.)
3 Dependent personality disorder. (Select two options.)

111

Disorders of sexual preference

Options:

- (a) Reliance on some non-living object as a stimulus for sexual arousal and sexual gratification.
- (b) The wearing of clothes of the opposite sex principally to obtain sexual excitement.
- (c) A recurrent or persistent tendency to expose the genitalia to strangers without inviting or intending closer contact.
- (d) A recurrent or persistent tendency to look at people engaging in sexual or intimate behaviour such as undressing.
- (e) A sexual preference for children, usually of prepubertal or early pubertal age.
- (f) A preference for sexual activity that involves bondage or the infliction of pain or humiliation.
- (g) Interest in rubbing, usually one's pelvic area or erect penis, against a non-consenting person for sexual pleasure.

Match the diagnoses below with their descriptions, from the above.

1 Frotteurism
2 Fetishistic transvestism
3 Fetishism
4 Sadomasochism

Diagnosis

Options:

- (a) Borderline personality disorder
- (b) Early-onset dementia
- (c) Hypochondriacal disorder
- (d) Antisocial personality disorder
- (e) Generalised anxiety disorder
- (f) Dissociative fugue
- (g) Somatisation disorder
- (h) No diagnosis

Select the most likely diagnosis for each of the vignettes below from the list above. (Only one diagnosis applies to each vignette.)

1 A 22-year-old man is preoccupied with the idea he has stomach cancer. He has had several investigations that rule it out, but he is difficult to reassure. He seems to eventually accept that he does not have this condition and instead insists he has bowel cancer. His mood is low and he is very anxious, but he does not fulfil criteria for a diagnosis of depressive or anxiety disorder.

2 A 33-year-old woman is referred to a psychiatry out-patient clinic. She has had a number of gastrointestinal symptoms for several years,

and also aches and pains in her joints. Both have been investigated intensively and no cause has been found. You are the fourteenth doctor she has seen in the past 2 years.

3 A 45-year-old goes missing from his place of work in London for several days. Family members who live close by have not seen him in over a week. Some days later, he is found by police in the north of Scotland, where his late mother was from. He had been under enormous pressure at work. He has no recollection of the episode. He did not engage in any untoward behaviour during his trip.

MCQ answers

1 Which of the following is not true of behaviours in personality disorder according to ICD-10?
   (a) An enduring pattern that deviates markedly from the culturally expected range
   (b) Occurs across a broad range of personal and social situations
   (c) Causes personal distress
   (d) **Onset is in early adulthood**
   (e) Is inflexible, maladaptive, or otherwise dysfunctional

As well as the specific behaviours and symptoms identified by ICD-10 to categorise specific personality disorders, there are a set of general criteria required for diagnosis. One of these is evidence that the behavioural problems are stable and of long duration, having onset in late childhood or adolescence. Personality disorders are likely to be reclassified in ICD-11: under the proposed classification, it will be possible to diagnose personality disorder at any age. See Tyrer *et al* (2011) and WHO (1992).

2 An 18-year-old woman presents to the emergency department with superficial, self-inflicted cuts to her arms. She said that she did this to relieve tension, as she has been feeling very low in mood and does not have hope for the future. However, her mother says that earlier in the day she seemed to be in a good mood and was laughing with her in the kitchen. When they later argued, she became very angry and began to scream at her mother, saying that no one loved her. She has a very unstable relationship with her boyfriend and she is preoccupied with her weight and uncertain about her sexuality. What is the most likely diagnosis here?
   (a) Depression
   (b) Bipolar disorder
   (c) **Emotionally unstable personality disorder**
   (d) Anorexia nervosa
   (e) Schizoid personality disorder

This woman probably fulfils ICD-10 criteria for a diagnosis of emotionally unstable personality disorder (EUPD), borderline type (the DSM-5 equivalent is borderline personality disorder). Individuals with this disorder experience a lot of distress throughout their teenage and adult lives and have fractious and often volatile difficult relationships with others. They have unstable and capricious moods. Comorbid depression is common, although in this case the patient's mood does not seem to have been low for an extended period prior to the incident. Problems with self-image and sexuality are frequently seen. Self-harm is also common but, as NICE guidelines stress, this should not be used on its own to diagnose EUPD.

The cause of EUPD is unclear, but an interaction between biological (e.g. temperamental) and psychosocial (e.g. adverse childhood events) factors probably provides the best explanation for how the condition develops. Patients with EUPD report many negative events (e.g. trauma, neglect) during childhood and have high rates of childhood sexual abuse. See Cowen *et al* (2012) and WHO (1992) and, for further reading, Kendall *et al* (2009) and Leichsenring *et al* (2011).

3   Anankastic personality disorder shares some characteristics with which other psychiatric disorder?
   (a)   Generalised anxiety disorder
   (b)   Panic disorder
   (c)   PTSD
   (d)   Agoraphobia
   (e)   **OCD**

Anankastic (obsessive–compulsive) personality disorder is characterised by feelings of excessive doubt and caution, preoccupation with details, order and schedule, excessive conscientiousness and scrupulousness, pedantry, adherence to social conventions, and unreasonable insistence that others submit to exactly their way of doing things. Intrusion of insistent and unwelcome thoughts or impulses is also a feature.

Patients with this disorder share certain features with individuals with OCD, although the precise nature of the relationship between the two is contentious. One of the key differences at a clinical level is the experience of obsessive and compulsive behaviours: to those with anankastic personality disorder, they are egosyntonic (in keeping with their view of the world and do not cause distress), whereas in OCD, they are egodystonic (unwanted and seen as unhealthy and the product of anxiety-inducing and involuntary thoughts). See WHO (1992) and, for further reading, Mancebo *et al* (2005).

4   A 34-year-old man is referred to the out-patient clinic, reporting ongoing difficulties with his landlord. He has been in several arguments with him and says that his landlord is to blame for these. He admits that he drinks late into the night, but denies his landlord's accusations that he is playing loud music and shouting. He has several arrests for assaults and has been violent to previous girlfriends, with whom he has only had short-term relationships. He does not understand why his last girlfriend was upset when he hit her. What type of personality disorder does this man have?

   (a)   Schizoid
   (b)   **Dissocial/antisocial**
   (c)   Schizotypal
   (d)   Emotionally unstable
   (e)   Narcissistic

This man has dissocial personality disorder, according to ICD-10 criteria (the DSM-5 equivalent is antisocial personality disorder). It is marked by callous and non-empathic behaviour towards other people, negative attitudes towards rules and social norms and an inability to maintain enduring relationships. Individuals with this condition often have criminal convictions and become involved in violent altercations.

Although not a recognised condition in the major classificatory manuals, experts in the field deem psychopathy to be a severe form of dissocial/antisocial personality disorder. Psychopathy is assessed using the Hare Psychopathy Checklist. Both antisocial/dissocial personality disorder and psychopathy are thought to involve an interplay of environmental and neurobiological factors. Dysregulation of the limbic system and prefrontal cortex has been repeatedly implicated. See Hare & Vertommen (2003) and WHO (1992) and, for further reading, Glenn & Raine (2011).

5   A 22-year-old university student is referred by his GP as she is concerned that he might be psychotic. He spends hours each day playing computer games and watching fantasy epic films and programmes. He speaks a lot about characters from these programmes and how he relates to them. He does not have any close friends or intimate relationships. He dresses in a strange, dishevelled manner and is not responsive to concerns expressed by peers and lecturers about his personal hygiene. His mother says that he was an odd, withdrawn child who showed little affection for his siblings and that his behaviour has not changed in recent years. On assessment, the psychiatrist feels that he has a personality disorder, rather than psychosis. What disorder does he diagnose?

   (a)   Antisocial
   (b)   **Schizoid**
   (c)   Schizotypal
   (d)   Emotionally unstable
   (e)   Narcissistic

Although this man has some features that resemble negative symptoms of schizophrenia, his overall presentation is more in keeping with a diagnosis of schizoid personality disorder. This condition is characterised by a lack of interest in social relationships, a tendency towards a solitary lifestyle, secretiveness, and emotional coldness and apathy. However, affected individuals can simultaneously demonstrate a rich, elaborate and exclusively internal fantasy world.

The diagnosis has come under scrutiny in recent times, with some authors contending that schizoid individuals actually fall into two distinct groups: an affect-constricted group, which might better be subsumed within schizotypal personality disorder, and a seclusive group, which might better be subsumed within avoidant personality disorder. However, this is not yet a clinical guideline. Other research suggests genetic links with conditions such as schizophrenia and Asperger's syndrome. See WHO (1992) and, for further reading, Mittal *et al* (2007) and Triebwasser *et al* (2012).

6   Which of the following is not a core feature of schizotypal disorder?

   (a)   Inappropriate or constricted affect
   (b)   Behaviour or appearance that is odd, eccentric, or peculiar
   (c)   Poor rapport with others and a tendency to social withdrawal
   (d)   **Inability to maintain enduring relationships, although no difficulty in establishing them**
   (e)   Occasional quasi-psychotic episodes with illusions, hallucinations, and delusion-like ideas

Schizotypal disorder (schizotypal personality disorder in DSM-5) is grouped with schizophrenia and other psychotic disorders in ICD-10. This reflects the conceptualisation of the condition by many as a 'schizophrenia spectrum disorder'. Schizotypal disorder is far more common in relatives of individuals with schizophrenia than in relatives of people with other mental illnesses or in people without mentally ill relatives.

Patients with schizotypal disorder and patients with chronic schizophrenia share cognitive, social, and attentional deficits hypothesised to result from common neurodevelopmental pathology. However, these deficits are milder in patients with schizotypal disorder, which is thought to be because other, related brain regions are recruited to compensate for dysfunctional areas. See WHO (1992) and, for further reading, Chemerinski *et al* (2013).

7   A 20-year-old student is referred to your clinic because of her GP's concerns about her weight loss. She has lost several kilograms in recent weeks and her BMI is now 16.5. She is continuing to attend university and sees no problem with her weight. In fact she believes she should lose more as she is 'still a bit fat'. She has stopped having periods. Which of the following features are not supportive of a diagnosis of anorexia nervosa?

   (a)   Self-induced vomiting and purging
   (b)   Excessive exercise
   (c)   Use of appetite suppressants and diuretics
   (d)   **Dark hair on arms and legs**
   (e)   Preoccupation with food

As well as the core ICD-10 features of anorexia nervosa – weight loss of $> 15\%$ (or BMI $< 17.5 \, \text{kg/m}^2$), avoidance of 'fattening' foods, morbid fear of fatness, endocrine dysfunction resulting in amenorrhoea in females (or loss of sexual interest in males) – there are several other features that support the diagnosis. One of these is lanugo: very fine, soft and usually unpigmented downy hair growing on the face and body. See Semple & Smyth (2013a) and WHO (1992).

8   A 45-year-old teacher is having difficulty at work. He believes his colleagues are plotting against him and that they wish to force him to leave his job. He has had confrontations with several colleagues in which he has cited human rights law, and has threatened to use a solicitor. When one colleague asked him about his weekend plans, he was convinced this meant she was suggesting that he clear out his desk. He believes that it is right that he be promoted to vice-principal as he is clearly the best teacher in the school. He has left or been asked to leave four previous schools because of similar problems. What is the likely diagnosis?

     (a)   Antisocial personality disorder
     (b)   Schizophrenia
     (c)   Delusional disorder
     (d)   **Paranoid personality disorder**
     (e)   Narcissistic personality disorder

Paranoid personality disorder is characterised by suspiciousness and a pervasive tendency to distort experience by misconstruing the neutral or friendly actions of others as hostile, a tendency to bear grudges persistently, a combative and tenacious sense of personal rights out of keeping with the actual situation, a tendency to experience excessive self-importance, and a preoccupation with unsubstantiated 'conspiratorial' explanations of events both immediate to the patient and in the world at large. Such individuals are highly querulous and often cause serious disruption in the workplace or the community. Their reduced capacity for meaningful emotional involvement and the general pattern of isolation overlaps with the other DSM-5 Cluster A personality disorders.

A recent review pointed out that there is comparatively little published evidence for the reliability and validity of paranoid personality disorder and called for its exclusion from future diagnostic manuals. It has been excluded from Section III of DSM-5, which identifies disorders for further research. See Triebwasser *et al* (2013) and WHO (1992) and, for further reading, Harper (2010).

9　An underweight 19-year-old woman with a BMI of $16\,kg/m^2$, and a history of self-induced vomiting, dietary restriction and a morbid fear of fatness presents to an out-patient clinic. Which of the following psychological treatments is not recommended in the NICE guidelines for treatment of her condition?

(a)　**Psychoanalysis**
(b)　Cognitive–behavioural therapy
(c)　Interpersonal psychotherapy
(d)　Cognitive analytic therapy
(e)　Family interventions focused explicitly on eating disorders

According to NICE, therapies to be considered for the psychological treatment of anorexia nervosa include cognitive analytic therapy, cognitive–behavioural therapy, interpersonal psychotherapy, and family interventions focused explicitly on eating disorders. Patient and, where appropriate, carer preference should be taken into account when deciding on the psychological treatment. However, a word of caution is required here. A 2007 systematic review concluded that the evidence for effective treatments of anorexia nervosa is limited, a view supported by all Cochrane reviews to date. See Bulik *et al* (2007), NICE (2004), WHO (1992) and, for further reading, the Cochrane library.

10　A 25-year-old accountant attends your out-patient clinic, reporting low mood. When you explore her story, it becomes clear that food plays a very important role in her life. She speaks of craving food a lot of the time and describes binging on large amounts of cake and chocolates, often alone in her room. She admits that sometimes she induces vomiting. She is of normal weight but feels she is too fat. Which pharmacological treatment is indicated for her condition?

(a)　Tricyclic antidepressant
(b)　**SSRI**
(c)　First-generation antipsychotic
(d)　Second-generation antipsychotic
(e)　Benzodiazepine

This woman has bulimia nervosa. SSRIs, specifically fluoxetine, are the first-choice pharmacological treatment for bulimia nervosa in terms of acceptability, tolerability and reduction of symptoms. The effective dose of fluoxetine for bulimia nervosa (60 mg daily) is higher than that used for depression. No medications, other than antidepressants, are recommended for the treatment of bulimia nervosa. Fluoxetine decreases the core symptoms of binge eating and purging and associated psychological features in the short term, whereas cognitive–behavioural therapy reduces core behavioural and psychological features in the short and long term. See NICE (2004) and, for further reading, Shapiro *et al* (2007).

11 The mother of a 21-year-old woman attending your clinic asks to meet you. She is worried that her daughter has an eating disorder. She had some problems with binge-eating when she was younger. Which of the following is true about eating disorders?

(a) They are more common in males than females
(b) Genetic factors are not important
(c) **Environmental factors are important**
(d) They are more common in low-income countries
(e) They do not affect mortality

Environmental factors play a large role in the development of eating disorders. Idealisation of thinness, resulting weight concerns and personality factors such as negative emotionality and perfectionism have been shown to contribute significantly. Genetic factors are also important, and twin and family studies derive high heritability estimates; however, causal genetic mechanisms are as yet unidentified. Eating disorders are much more common in females than males, with a ratio of approximately 7:1.

Recent studies demonstrate that eating disorders and abnormal eating behaviours do occur in non-Western countries and among ethnic minorities, although they are less common. The increasing prevalence of eating disorders in non-Western countries has been associated with cultural transition and globalisation, including modernisation, urbanisation and exposure to media promoting the Western beauty-ideal. All eating disorders have an elevated mortality risk; anorexia nervosa has the highest risk, with a standardised mortality ratio (ratio of observed deaths in the study population to expected deaths in the population of origin) of 5.9 reported in one major study. See Cowen *et al* (2012) and, for further reading, Hinney & Volckmar (2013), Keel & Forney (2013) and Smink *et al* (2012).

12 A 35-year-old businessman enjoys dressing up in his wife's clothes. He says he does so to experience what it feels like to be a woman and it does not cause him sexual arousal. He has no desire to be a woman. What is the correct term to describe his behaviour?

(a) Transsexualism
(b) **Dual-role transvestism**
(c) Fetishism
(d) Fetishistic transvestism
(e) Exhibitionism

Transvestism refers to cross-dressing. Dual-role transvestism is defined by ICD-10 as wearing clothes of the opposite sex in order to experience temporary membership of the opposite sex, with the absence of any sexual motivation for the cross-dressing and the absence of any desire to change permanently into the opposite sex. In fetishistic transvestism, cross-dressing is closely associated with sexual arousal. Once orgasm occurs and sexual arousal declines, there is a strong desire to remove the clothing.

Transsexualism, on the other hand, refers to a desire to live and be accepted as a member of the opposite sex, usually accompanied by the wish to make one's body as congruent as possible with one's preferred sex through surgery and hormonal treatment. Both transvestism and transsexualism are categorised under gender identity disorders in ICD-10, although this term is controversial and has been replaced by gender dysphoria in DSM-5. See WHO (1992) and, for further reading, APA (2013) and Moran (2013).

13 A 34-year-old man is involved in a minor road accident. He has a small bruise on his neck but no pain or dysfunction. He tells his wife he is hoping to get a payout from his insurance company. He tells his GP he has severe back pain and PTSD and is referred to you for assessment. What is the correct term to describe his behaviour?

  (a)   Factitious disorder (Munchausen's syndrome)
  (b)   **Malingering**
  (c)   Conversion disorder
  (d)   Somatoform disorder
  (e)   Elaboration of physical symptoms for psychological reasons

This man is malingering. He is clearly falsifying his symptoms for a secondary gain: in this case, compensation. His motivation is not psychological, or, as in the case of factitious disorder, for the primary purpose of gaining medical assessment and treatment.

Assessing the malingering of psychological symptoms is very difficult, and remains a contentious issue. However, considerable research has led to the development of more robust formal assessments. A detailed history and focus on the consistency of symptoms and problems remains an important aspect of assessment. See WHO (1992) and, for further reading, Jelicic *et al* (2011) and Rogers (2008).

14 A 56-year-old woman spends half of her weekly budget on gaming scratch cards. She makes small wins but ultimately loses financially each week. She has repeatedly tried to stop doing this but has failed. It causes her a lot of distress as she is not well off and it also interrupts her working and leisure routine. She has intrusive thoughts about buying scratch cards when she is at work. What is her diagnosis?

  (a)   Trichotillomania
  (b)   **Pathological gambling**
  (c)   No diagnosis
  (d)   Kleptomania
  (e)   Other habit and impulse disorder

This woman has a diagnosis of pathological gambling, which is classified in ICD-10 as a habit and impulse disorder. Gambling can wreak havoc on the lives of people affected, their families and society. Common social costs include negative effects on gamblers' physical and mental health and performance in vocational situations, and hardship (via debts and asset losses) that can lead to legal consequences, such as bankruptcy, loans, or criminal acts to gain money. Costs imposed on society include the cost of crimes committed by some gamblers and costs related to their treatment.

There is some contention about the clinical validity of habit and impulse disorder diagnoses. However, neurobiological research has shown the potential involvement of serotonergic, dopaminergic and opioid dysfunction in the pathophysiology of pathological gambling and other habit and impulse disorders. Experimental treatment strategies for pathological gambling include pharmacological options such as SSRIs, opioid receptor antagonists, anti-addiction drugs and mood stabilisers, and also psychological interventions such as cognitive–behavioural therapy. See Raylu & Oei (2002) and, for further reading, Brewer & Potenza (2008) and Iancu *et al* (2008).

EMI answers

Personality disorder traits

Options:

- (a) Self-dramatisation
- (b) Excessive preoccupation with being criticised or rejected in social situations
- (c) Unwillingness to become involved with people unless certain of being liked
- (d) Encouraging or allowing others to make most of one's own important life decisions
- (e) Subordination of one's own needs to those of others on whom one is dependent
- (f) Continual seeking for excitement and activities in which the patient is the centre of attention
- (g) Inappropriate seductiveness in appearance or behaviour
- (h) Restrictions in lifestyle because of need to have physical security

The items above are traits of which personality disorder? (More than one item for each answer below.)

1 Histrionic personality disorder

(a) Self-dramatisation

(f) Continual seeking for excitement and activities in which the patient is the centre of attention

(g) Inappropriate seductiveness in appearance or behaviour

2 Anxious/avoidant personality disorder

(b) Excessive preoccupation with being criticised or rejected in social situations

(c) Unwillingness to become involved with people unless certain of being liked

(h) Restrictions in lifestyle because of need to have physical security

3 Dependent personality disorder

(d) Encouraging or allowing others to make most of one's own important life decisions

(e) Subordination of one's own needs to those of others on whom one is dependent

Disorders of sexual preference

Options:

- (a) Reliance on some non-living object as a stimulus for sexual arousal and sexual gratification
- (b) The wearing of clothes of the opposite sex principally to obtain sexual excitement
- (c) A recurrent or persistent tendency to expose the genitalia to strangers without inviting or intending closer contact
- (d) A recurrent or persistent tendency to look at people engaging in sexual or intimate behaviour such as undressing
- (e) A sexual preference for children, usually of prepubertal or early pubertal age
- (f) A preference for sexual activity that involves bondage or the infliction of pain or humiliation
- (g) Interest in rubbing, usually one's pelvic area or erect penis, against a non-consenting person for sexual pleasure

Match the diagnoses below with their descriptions, from the above.

1 Frotteurism

(g) Interest in rubbing, usually one's pelvic area or erect penis, against a non-consenting person for sexual pleasure

2 Fetishistic transvestism

(b) The wearing of clothes of the opposite sex principally to obtain sexual excitement

3 Fetishism

(a) Reliance on some non-living object as a stimulus for sexual arousal and sexual gratification

4 Sadomasochism

(f) A preference for sexual activity that involves bondage or the infliction of pain or humiliation

Diagnosis

Options:

- (a) Borderline personality disorder
- (b) Early-onset dementia
- (c) Hypochondriacal disorder
- (d) Antisocial personality disorder
- (e) Generalised anxiety disorder
- (f) Dissociative fugue
- (g) Somatisation disorder
- (h) No diagnosis

Select the most likely diagnosis for each of the vignettes below from the list above. (Only one diagnosis applies to each vignette.)

1   A 22-year-old man is preoccupied with the idea he has stomach cancer. He has had several investigations that rule it out, but he is difficult to reassure. He seems to eventually accept that he does not have this condition and instead insists he has bowel cancer. His mood is low and he is very anxious, but he does not fulfil criteria for a diagnosis of depressive or anxiety disorder.

(c) Hypochondriacal disorder

2   A 33-year-old woman is referred to a psychiatry out-patient clinic. She has had a number of gastrointestinal symptoms for several years, and also aches and pains in her joints. Both have been investigated intensively and no cause has been found. You are the fourteenth doctor she has seen in the past 2 years.

(g) Somatisation disorder

3   A 45-year-old goes missing from his place of work in London for several days. Family members who live close by have not seen him in over a week. Some days later, he is found by police in the north of Scotland, where his late mother was from. He had been under enormous pressure at work. He has no recollection of the episode. He did not engage in any untoward behaviour during his trip.

(f) Dissociative fugue

Physical health in psychiatry and functional somatic disorders

---

MCQs

1 A young man, recently diagnosed with schizophrenia, has a 5-year history of cigarette smoking. Which of the following is true?

   (a) The prevalence of smoking in patients with schizophrenia is the same as in the general population

   (b) The majority of smokers with schizophrenia don't wish to stop smoking

   (c) Smoking can alter the metabolism of antipsychotics

   (d) Smoking has no impact on mental health

   (e) People with schizophrenia don't have higher rates of smoking-related illness

2 A 35-year-old female patient with a diagnosis of schizophrenia attends the clinic concerned that her GP informed her that she has metabolic syndrome. All the following are part of the metabolic syndrome, except:

   (a) Raised HDL cholesterol

   (b) Raised triglyceride levels

   (c) Raised blood pressure

   (d) Increased waist circumference

   (e) Raised fasting glucose

3 A 25-year-old woman was recently started on antipsychotic treatment combined with cognitive–behavioural therapy for a first episode of psychosis. She has been treated with the antipsychotic for 2 months and attends the clinic reporting increased appetite and weight gain. Which of the following antipsychotics are most associated with weight gain?

   (a) Amisulpride

   (b) Aripiprazole

   (c) Haloperidol

   (d) Olanzapine

   (e) Paliperidone

4 You are working as a psychiatry senior house officer in a community mental health team. Because of the high rates of patient obesity you observe in your clinic, you establish a physical health monitoring clinic. Which of the following is true?

(a) Psychiatrists should not diagnose and treat physical illnesses
(b) Physical health complaints need not be prioritised
(c) A lack of integration of psychiatry and general medical settings does not impact on physical healthcare
(d) Monitoring for cardiovascular risk factors in psychiatry is adequate
(e) Iatrogenic factors account for considerable physical morbidity

5 A 50-year-old woman attends the psychiatry out-patient clinic after a recent general hospital admission for complications secondary to a medical disorder. All the following have increased prevalence in severe mental illnesses, except:

(a) Cardiovascular disease
(b) Diabetes mellitus
(c) Rheumatoid arthritis
(d) Hepatitis B
(e) Osteoporosis

6 A 45-year-old woman with paranoid schizophrenia has become concerned about her physical health and asks you for advice. All the following are patient-related factors that increase physical health morbidity, except:

(a) Good family support
(b) Active symptoms of psychosis limiting ability to attend to physical healthcare
(c) Lifestyle factors
(d) Difficulty comprehending medical advice
(e) Difficulty in communicating physical health needs

7 At your multidisciplinary team meeting, you and your colleagues discuss ways to address the high rate of physical morbidity in your patient group. The increased physical morbidity associated with severe mental illnesses might be contributed to by all the following clinician-related factors, except:

(a) Stigmatisation
(b) Physical complaints regarded as psychosomatic symptoms
(c) Beliefs that patients will not adopt healthy lifestyle recommendations
(d) Paying equal attention to mental and physical health symptoms
(e) Decreased knowledge regarding medical issues among psychiatrists

8   A 35-year-old man with a 10-year history of psychotic illness attends the clinic seeking advice on lifestyle changes. He is concerned that unhealthy lifestyle habits might be putting his physical health at risk. Which of the following is true of mortality and life expectancy in psychotic disorders?

(a)   Life expectancy is reduced by 15–20 years in comparison with the general population
(b)   Life expectancy is the same as that for the general population
(c)   Any reduction in life expectancy is largely explained by an increased rate of suicide
(d)   Cardiovascular disease does not excessively contribute to mortality
(e)   Death rates from cancer are lower in comparison with the general population

9   A patient with schizophrenia, treated with clozapine, has developed type 2 diabetes. Which of the following would be a recommended first-line pharmacological intervention for type 2 diabetes in this case?

(a)   Switch to aripiprazole
(b)   Metformin
(c)   Insulin
(d)   Methylphenidate
(e)   Fluoxetine

10   A physical health monitoring service is offered in your clinic as part of ongoing follow-up for patients with psychotic illnesses. Which of the following is the least likely parameter to be measured in people with psychotic illness?

(a)   Blood pressure
(b)   Fasting glucose
(c)   Serum cholesterol
(d)   Serum triglycerides
(e)   Waist circumference

11   A patient you assess at your clinic with a diagnosis of schizophrenia was recently treated for a myocardial infarction. You speak to your consultant about cardiovascular risk factors in patients with schizophrenia. Which of the following is the most prevalent modifiable cardiovascular risk factor in patients with schizophrenia?

(a)   Cigarette smoking
(b)   Hypertension
(c)   Dyslipidaemia
(d)   Obesity
(e)   Type 2 diabetes

12 A 26-year-old male patient with treatment-resistant schizophrenia has recently begun treatment with clozapine. Some 4 weeks into treatment, he presents with thirst, increased urination, fatigue, loss of appetite, nausea and vomiting. Which of the following is the most likely diagnosis?

   (a)   Infection secondary to neutropenia
   (b)   Myocarditis
   (c)   Diabetic ketoacidosis
   (d)   Hyperthyroidism
   (e)   Pneumonia

13 A 20-year-old woman with a diagnosis of anorexia nervosa attends an emergency out-patient review. She collapsed at home earlier that day. All the following are medical indications for admission in anorexia nervosa, except:

   (a)   BMI of $<18\,kg/m^2$
   (b)   Hypokalaemia
   (c)   Bradycardia ($<40\,bpm$)
   (d)   Petechial rash and platelet suppression
   (e)   Hypoglycaemia

14 A 19-year-old woman is referred to the clinic by a neurologist. She was initially assessed by the neurologist for epilepsy, but a diagnosis of non-epileptic seizures has been made. All the following would suggest that the woman is presenting with non-epileptic seizures, except:

   (a)   Thrashing movements
   (b)   Seizure episode lasting longer than 5 min
   (c)   Eyes closed during seizure episode
   (d)   Side-to-side head shaking
   (e)   Sudden onset

15 A 33-year-old woman attends an out-patient assessment. She has been experiencing persistent fatigue for the past 3 years and is concerned that she might have chronic fatigue syndrome. Which of the following symptoms would most support this diagnosis?

   (a)   Post-exertion fatigue
   (b)   Loss of appetite
   (c)   Early morning wakening
   (d)   Loss of libido
   (e)   Diurnal variation in fatigue

16 You are called to review a 70-year-old woman on a medical ward who has been confused since the time of her admission. The nurse on duty tells you that she is displaying evidence of dementia, even though there is no documented history of cognitive impairment. The following features are all more commonly found in delirium than in dementia, except:

(a) Lability of affect
(b) Insidious onset
(c) Restlessness
(d) Inattention
(e) Visual hallucination

17 A 75-year-old woman, who was hospitalised 3 days ago, presents with delirium. All the following are risk factors for the development of delirium, except:

(a) Hearing impairment
(b) Concurrent infection
(c) Dehydration
(d) Family history of delirium
(e) Pain

18 A 45-year-old male patient with depression attends the out-patient clinic. He presents with features of atypical depression. Which of the following symptoms would you be likely find in such a presentation?

(a) Insomnia
(b) Weight gain
(c) Agitation
(d) Early morning wakening
(e) Mood elevation

19 A 22-year-old woman attends the clinic with a 1-month history of low mood. She was diagnosed with epilepsy 6 months previously and is concerned about the risk of developing mental illness. The prevalence of all the following disorders is increased in epilepsy, except:

(a) Depression
(b) Suicide
(c) Psychosis
(d) Dementia
(e) Anxiety

EMI questions

Clinical investigations

Options:

(a) Full blood count
(b) Electrocardiogram
(c) Waist circumference
(d) Fasting serum glucose
(e) Thyroid function tests
(f) Creatine kinase
(g) Serum creatinine
(h) Serum prolactin

Select one investigation from the above list that would be recommended for each of the following clinical scenarios.

1   A 40-year-old woman was started on clozapine 4 weeks ago. It is necessary that this investigation is performed and results be normal before her prescription of clozapine can be fulfilled.

2   A 22-year-old man with a diagnosis of schizophrenia and with a family history of diabetes is reporting sexual dysfunction while treated with risperidone.

3   A 35-year-old woman was admitted with a manic episode with psychotic features. She has been treated with intramuscular haloperidol for the past 3 days because of high levels of agitation and refusal to adhere with oral medication. She presents with a temperature of 38.5 °C, confusion and muscle rigidity.

Treatment interventions

Options:

(a) Start aripiprazole
(b) Start metformin
(c) Diet and exercise plan
(d) Start atorvastatin
(e) Stop clozapine
(f) Start depot medication
(g) Start antidepressant medication
(h) Start methylphenidate

Select two interventions from the options above that would be recommended for each of the following clinical scenarios.

1   A 30-year-old man with a diagnosis of schizophrenia has remained stable while treated with olanzapine for the past 5 years. At his 6-monthly physical health check-up, he presents with two consecutive fasting serum glucose levels of 7.5 mmol/L (reference range 0–6.9 mmol/L) and has a HbA1c of 6.9% (52 mmol/mol) (reference range 4.0–5.9% (20–41 mmol/mol)).

2 A 32-year-old woman has been treated for the past 3 months with clozapine. She presents with weight gain. She has recently completed a diet and exercise programme but without any improvement in her weight.

3 A 36-year-old woman with schizophrenia has been stable while treated with clozapine for the past 10 years. At her 6-monthly physical health check-up, she has elevated serum cholesterol at 6.7 mmol/L (reference range 0–5.0 mmol/L) and an elevated low-density-lipoprotein cholesterol, at 4.1 mmol/L (reference range 0–3.0 mmol/L). This is the second occasion that she has had similar abnormal blood results.

MCQ answers

1 A young man, recently diagnosed with schizophrenia, has a 5-year history of cigarette smoking. Which of the following is true?

   (a) The prevalence of smoking in patients with schizophrenia is the same as in the general population
   (b) The majority of smokers with schizophrenia don't wish to stop smoking
   (c) **Smoking can alter the metabolism of antipsychotics**
   (d) Smoking has no impact on mental health
   (e) People with schizophrenia don't have higher rates of smoking-related illness

The rate of cigarette smoking is significantly higher in people with schizophrenia (and other psychotic disorders) compared with the general population. In the UK, 60% of those with psychotic disorders smoke, despite the significant reduction in smoking among the general population (39% in 1980 v. 20% in 2010). Furthermore, people with schizophrenia smoke more heavily and demonstrate greater levels of nicotine dependence compared with those without mental health problems.

Many people with schizophrenia wish to stop smoking, but are often overlooked in terms of nicotine replacement therapies and advice on smoking cessation. In the UK, up to 40% of all tobacco is smoked by people with mental health problems, yet these individuals are less likely than the general population to be offered support to quit.

Cigarette smoke contains polycyclic aromatic hydrocarbons, which can induce the metabolism of CYP 1A2 enzymes and increase the metabolism of certain medications, including clozapine, thus leading to lower serum levels. Smoking has been associated with a detrimental effect on mood and psychotic symptoms in schizophrenia and with heightened distress from psychotic-like experiences. See Van Gastel et al (2013).

2   A 35-year-old female patient with a diagnosis of schizophrenia attends the clinic concerned that her GP informed her that she has metabolic syndrome. All the following are part of the metabolic syndrome, except:

(a)   **Raised HDL cholesterol**
(b)   Raised triglyceride levels
(c)   Raised blood pressure
(d)   Increased waist circumference
(e)   Raised fasting glucose

It is estimated that 1/5–1/4 of the world's adults have this syndrome. Individuals meeting criteria for metabolic syndrome have a 3- to 6-fold increased risk of developing type 2 diabetes and a 2- to 6-fold risk of mortality due to cardiovascular disease. Metabolic syndrome is highly prevalent among treated patients with schizophrenia, with prevalence rates of 34–60%.

According to the new International Diabetes Federation definition, for a person to be diagnosed as having metabolic syndrome, they must have central obesity (defined for people of Europid origin as a waist circumference of ≥ 94 cm for men and ≥ 80 cm for women), plus two of the following four factors:

▶   raised triglycerides (≥ 1.7 mmol/L) or specific treatment for this lipid abnormality
▶   reduced HDL cholesterol (< 1.03 mmol/L in men and < 1.29 mmol/L in women) or specific treatment for this lipid abnormality
▶   raised systolic (≥ 130 mm Hg) or diastolic (≥ 85 mm Hg) blood pressure or treatment of previously diagnosed hypertension
▶   raised fasting plasma glucose (≥ 5.6 mmol/L) or previously diagnosed type 2 diabetes.

See Alberti *et al* (2006).

3   A 25-year-old woman was recently started on antipsychotic treatment combined with cognitive–behavioural therapy for a first episode of psychosis. She has been treated with the antipsychotic for 2 months and attends the clinic reporting increased appetite and weight gain. Which of the following antipsychotics are most associated with weight gain?

(a)   Amisulpride
(b)   Aripiprazole
(c)   Haloperidol
(d)   **Olanzapine**
(e)   Paliperidone

Olanzapine (along with clozapine) is associated with the greatest risk and degree of weight gain with antipsychotic treatment. Amisulpride and aripiprazole are considered weight-neutral antipsychotic medications. Haloperidol and paliperidone can have mild to moderate effects on weight gain. The initial weight gain over the first 6 weeks of antipsychotic treatment seems to be especially important, as patients do not tend to lose this weight later. See Bak *et al* (2014).

4   You are working as a psychiatry senior house officer in a community mental health team. Because of the high rates of patient obesity you observe in your clinic, you establish a physical health monitoring clinic. Which of the following is true?

(a)   Psychiatrists should not diagnose and treat physical illnesses
(b)   Physical health complaints need not be prioritised
(c)   A lack of integration of psychiatry and general medical settings does not impact on physical healthcare
(d)   Monitoring for cardiovascular risk factors in psychiatry is adequate
(e)   **Iatrogenic factors account for considerable physical morbidity**

Physical health monitoring is often overlooked in psychiatry. Iatrogenic factors in physical morbidity include the prescription of antipsychotic medications that can create or exacerbate cardiometabolic risk factors such as weight gain, dyslipidaemia and glucose dysregulation. There are also clinician- and service-related factors that affect physical morbidity, including lack of physician knowledge, negative attitudes, fragmented service organisation and social stigma ascribed to patients with severe mental illnesses. Lifestyle factors, which are relatively easy to measure, are frequently overlooked in screening, and baseline testing of important physical parameters is not sufficiently performed. See De Hert *et al* (2011*a*).

5   A 50-year-old woman attends the psychiatry out-patient clinic after a recent general hospital admission for complications secondary to a medical disorder. All the following have increased prevalence in severe mental illnesses, except:

(a)   Cardiovascular disease
(b)   Diabetes mellitus
(c)   **Rheumatoid arthritis**
(d)   Hepatitis B
(e)   Osteoporosis

All the above have increased prevalence rates in psychotic disorders, with the exception of rheumatoid arthritis, which is found at a reduced rate in schizophrenia. This finding was first reported as early as 1936. A variety of explanations have been put forward, including genetic factors and the anti-inflammatory effects of antipsychotic medication. See Leucht *et al* (2007).

6   A 45-year-old woman with paranoid schizophrenia has become concerned about her physical health and asks you for advice. All the following are patient-related factors that increase physical health morbidity, except:

(a)   **Good family support**
(b)   Active symptoms of psychosis limiting ability to attend to physical healthcare
(c)   Lifestyle factors
(d)   Difficulty comprehending medical advice
(e)   Difficulty in communicating physical health needs

Despite improved life expectancy rates in the general population, similar improvements have not been seen in people with severe mental illness. The increased mortality rates for people with severe mental illness are largely due to modifiable health factors, and this has led to calls for parity of physical and mental healthcare. An individual with a psychotic illness might have difficulty accessing and benefiting from medical care for many reasons: active symptoms of mental illness, cognitive difficulties, poor educational attainment, lifestyle factors (e.g. poor diet) and social isolation. People with good social networks and family relationships are more likely to benefit from assistance with medical treatment. See Leucht & Heres (2006).

7   At your multidisciplinary team meeting, you and your colleagues discuss ways to address the high rate of physical morbidity in your patient group. The increased physical morbidity associated with severe mental illnesses might be contributed to by all the following clinician-related factors, except:

(a)   Stigmatisation
(b)   Physical complaints regarded as psychosomatic symptoms
(c)   Beliefs that patients will not adopt healthy lifestyle recommendations
(d)   **Paying equal attention to mental and physical health symptoms**
(e)   Decreased knowledge regarding medical issues among psychiatrists

Except for answer (d), all the above are clinician-related factors that contribute to physical morbidity in severe mental illness. Unfortunately, these can be displayed by both psychiatrists and other doctors in their interactions with patients with mental illness. See De Hert *et al* (2011*a*).

8   A 35-year-old man with a 10-year history of psychotic illness attends the clinic seeking advice on lifestyle changes. He is concerned that unhealthy lifestyle habits might be putting his physical health at risk. Which of the following is true of mortality and life expectancy in psychotic disorders?

(a)   **Life expectancy is reduced by 15–20 years in comparison with the general population**
(b)   Life expectancy is the same as that for the general population
(c)   Any reduction in life expectancy is largely explained by an increased rate of suicide
(d)   Cardiovascular disease does not excessively contribute to mortality
(e)   Death rates from cancer are lower in comparison with the general population

People with severe mental illnesses, such as schizophrenia and bipolar affective disorder, have a higher risk of premature death, with mortality rates 2–3 times higher than in the general populations because of an increased risk of cardiovascular disease. This mortality gap, which has been widening in recent years, translates to a 15–20 years' shorter life expectancy once a diagnosis of serious mental illness is made. See Chang *et al* (2011).

9   A patient with schizophrenia, treated with clozapine, has developed type 2 diabetes. Which of the following would be a recommended first-line pharmacological intervention for type 2 diabetes in this case?

(a)   Switch to aripiprazole
(b)   **Metformin**
(c)   Insulin
(d)   Methylphenidate
(e)   Fluoxetine

Metformin would be an appropriate first-line treatment for type 2 diabetes in this case. Although the augmentation of clozapine with a more metabolically neutral antipsychotic (e.g. aripiprazole) might be beneficial for some, given that a diagnosis has been made, appropriate pharmacological treatment should be initiated (after considering non-pharmacological interventions). Metformin is also the first-choice medication to counteract antipsychotic-induced weight gain and other metabolic adverse effects in schizophrenia. See Mizuno *et al* (2014).

10 A physical health monitoring service is offered in your clinic as part of ongoing follow-up for patients with psychotic illnesses. Which of the following is the least likely parameter to be measured in people with psychotic illness?

   (a)   Blood pressure
   (b)   Fasting glucose
   (c)   Serum cholesterol
   (d)   Serum triglycerides
   (e)   **Waist circumference**

Waist circumference is the least frequently measured of the parameters in this question. It is also the most common abnormality of all metabolic syndrome criteria. BMI is another useful measure of obesity. Although BMI is relatively easy to assess, it is not monitored in over 50% of patients.

Increased waist circumference, indicating central obesity, is known to be closely associated with hyperinsulinaemia, dyslipidaemia and impaired glucose tolerance. It has been proposed that waist circumference or BMI alone could be used as a simple screening test for metabolic syndrome in schizophrenia. See Mitchell *et al* (2013).

11 A patient you assess at your clinic with a diagnosis of schizophrenia was recently treated for a myocardial infarction. You speak to your consultant about cardiovascular risk factors in patients with schizophrenia. Which of the following is the most prevalent modifiable cardiovascular risk factor in patients with schizophrenia?

   (a)   **Cigarette smoking**
   (b)   Hypertension
   (c)   Dyslipidaemia
   (d)   Obesity
   (e)   Type 2 diabetes

Cigarette smoking is the most common modifiable cardiovascular risk factor in patients with schizophrenia, with a prevalence of 50–80%. Hypertension is present in approximately 39% of people with schizophrenia, dyslipidaemia in 36–69%, obesity in 50–60% and type 2 diabetes in 10–15%. See De Hert *et al* (2011*b*) and Vancampfort *et al* (2015).

12 A 26-year-old male patient with treatment-resistant schizophrenia has recently begun treatment with clozapine. Some 4 weeks into treatment, he presents with thirst, increased urination, fatigue, loss of appetite, nausea and vomiting. Which of the following is the most likely diagnosis?

(a) Infection secondary to neutropenia
(b) Myocarditis
(c) **Diabetic ketoacidosis**
(d) Hyperthyroidism
(e) Pneumonia

Diabetic ketoacidosis is a medical emergency resulting from severe hyperglycaemia. The incidence of diabetic ketoacidosis for each second-generation (atypical) antipsychotic over a 7-year period is as follows: clozapine 2.2%; olanzapine 0.8%; and risperidone 0.2%. Onset of hyperglycaemia can be early in treatment, often occurring within 6 weeks of starting treatment. Most patients who develop diabetic ketoacidosis do not have pre-existing diabetes, but frequently have glucose dysregulation. See De Hert *et al* (2011*b*).

13 A 20-year-old woman with a diagnosis of anorexia nervosa attends an emergency out-patient review. She collapsed at home earlier that day. All the following are medical indications for admission in anorexia nervosa, except:

(a) **BMI of < 18 kg/m²**
(b) Hypokalaemia
(c) Bradycardia (< 40 bpm)
(d) Petechial rash and platelet suppression
(e) Hypoglycaemia

Medical indications for an admission include the following:

▶ BMI of < 13 kg/m² (or rapid decrease in weight (>1 kg/week))
▶ Syncope
▶ postural myopathy (assess with the stand-up–squat test)
▶ electrolyte imbalance (e.g. hypokalaemia K < 2.5 mmol/L, hyponatraemia Na< 125 mmol/L, hypophosphatemia PO_4< 0.5 mmol/L)
▶ hypoglycaemia (serum glucose < 2.5 mmol/L)
▶ petechial rash and platelet suppression (platelet count < 110 × 10⁹/L)
See Jones *et al* (2013).

14 A 19-year-old woman is referred to the clinic by a neurologist. She was initially assessed by the neurologist for epilepsy, but a diagnosis of non-epileptic seizures has been made. All the following would suggest that the woman is presenting with non-epileptic seizures, except:

(a) Thrashing movements
(b) Seizure episode lasting longer than 5 min
(c) Eyes closed during seizure episode
(d) Side-to-side head shaking
(e) **Sudden onset**

Movements during a 'thrashing' dissociative (non-epileptic) seizure are a form of severe tremor rather than clonic movements, and typically there is no isolated tonic phase. Dissociative seizures are more commonly associated with gradual rather than sudden onset, violent, thrashing movements, eyes and mouth closed during the episode (with eyes difficult to open), side-to-side head movements, prolonged seizure episode, recall for the period of unresponsiveness, and occasionally crying during or after the episode.

Incontinence of urine or faeces, tongue biting and pelvic thrusting, although less common in dissociative than epileptic seizures, can still occur, and are less helpful as distinguishing features. See Stone *et al* (2005).

15 A 33-year-old woman attends an out-patient assessment. She has been experiencing persistent fatigue for the past 3 years and is concerned that she might have chronic fatigue syndrome. Which of the following symptoms would most support this diagnosis?

    (a)   **Post-exertion fatigue**
    (b)   Loss of appetite
    (c)   Early morning wakening
    (d)   Loss of libido
    (e)   Diurnal variation in fatigue

For a diagnosis of chronic fatigue syndrome, a person must have at least 6 months of persistent fatigue that substantially reduces their level of activity. In addition, four or more of the following symptoms must occur in a 6-month period: impaired memory or concentration, sore throat, tender glands, aching or stiff muscles, multi-joint pain, new headaches, unrefreshing sleep, and post-exertion fatigue. Medical conditions that might explain the prolonged fatigue as well as a number of psychiatric diagnoses (eating disorders, psychotic disorders, bipolar disorder, depression and substance misuse within 2 years of the onset of fatigue) exclude a diagnosis of chronic fatigue syndrome. The other answers listed are symptoms of depression.

No single causal factor has been identified for chronic fatigue syndrome. Yet there are indications that infections and immunological dysfunction contribute to development and maintenance of symptoms, probably interacting with genetic and psychosocial factors. See Afari & Buchwald (2003) and Fukuda *et al* (1994).

16 You are called to review a 70-year-old woman on a medical ward who has been confused since the time of her admission. The nurse on duty tells you that she is displaying evidence of dementia, even though there is no documented history of cognitive impairment. The following features are all more commonly found in delirium than in dementia, except:

    (a)   Lability of affect
    (b)   **Insidious onset**
    (c)   Restlessness
    (d)   Inattention
    (e)   Visual hallucination

This woman is more likely to be experiencing delirium than dementia. Delirium is characterised by cognitive and neuropsychiatric symptoms in which inattention and reduced awareness are central. Delirium is of acute onset, fluctuates and occurs in the context of physical morbidity. Dementia, on the other hand, is characterised by a gradual, insidious onset of decline in memory and other cognitive abilities, such as planning and organizing, and the general processing of information. A gradual deterioration in activities of daily living is also seen.

Preserved awareness of the environment (i.e. absence of clouding of consciousness) distinguishes dementia from delirium. Evidence of damage to other higher cortical functions, such as aphasia, agnosia, or apraxia, is also a sign of dementia rather than delirium. See WHO (1992).

17 A 75-year-old woman, who was hospitalised 3 days ago, presents with delirium. All the following are risk factors for the development of delirium, except:
- (a) Hearing impairment
- (b) Concurrent infection
- (c) Dehydration
- (d) **Family history of delirium**
- (e) Pain

Delirium in a hospital setting is multifactorial. Causes include patient-related factors (age ≥ 70 years, pre-existing cognitive impairment, previous episode of delirium, number and severity of comorbid illnesses, hearing impairment, alcohol or drug dependence), illness-related factors (illness severity, concurrent infection, dehydration, fracture, hypoxia, metabolic/electrolyte disturbance, pain), procedural factors (surgery, longer duration of operation, catheterisation, emergency procedure) and medication-related factors (addition of ≥3 new medications, benzodiazepine use, anticholinergic use). See O'Connell *et al* (2014).

18 A 45-year-old male patient with depression attends the out-patient clinic. He presents with features of atypical depression. Which of the following symptoms would you be likely find in such a presentation?
- (a) Insomnia
- (b) **Weight gain**
- (c) Agitation
- (d) Early morning wakening
- (e) Mood elevation

Features of atypical depression include weight gain and increased appetite. Both depression and obesity are associated with various chronic diseases such as diabetes mellitus, hypertension, dyslipidaemia, cancer, and respiratory and osteoarticular diseases. Obesity could also be an explanation for the approximately doubled risk of cardiovascular disease and cerebrovascular diseases and the increased mortality among individuals with depression. See Lasserre *et al* (2014).

19 A 22-year-old woman attends the clinic with a 1-month history of low mood. She was diagnosed with epilepsy 6 months previously and is concerned about the risk of developing mental illness. The prevalence of all the following disorders is increased in epilepsy, except:

(a) Depression
(b) Suicide
(c) Psychosis
(d) **Dementia**
(e) Anxiety

Epilepsy is associated with an increased prevalence of neuropsychiatric disorders, with a reported prevalence of 30%. A clinician must identify if the psychiatric symptoms are related to the occurrence of seizures (pre-ictal, ictal, post-ictal), if they are related to the use of anticonvulsants or if the onset of symptoms is associated with the remission of seizures in patients who had previously failed to respond to anticonvulsants. Depression is found in 25–60% of those with epilepsy and the rate of suicide is increased by 2.4 compared with the general population. See Agrawal & Govender (2011).

EMI answers

Clinical investigations

Options:

(a) Full blood count
(b) Electrocardiogram
(c) Waist circumference
(d) Fasting serum glucose
(e) Thyroid function tests
(f) Creatine kinase
(g) Serum creatinine
(h) Serum prolactin

Select one investigation from the above list that would be recommended for each of the following clinical scenarios.

1   A 40-year-old woman was started on clozapine 4 weeks ago. It is necessary that this investigation is performed and results be normal before her prescription of clozapine can be fulfilled.
   (a) Full blood count

2   A 22-year-old man with a diagnosis of schizophrenia and with a family history of diabetes is reporting sexual dysfunction while treated with risperidone.
   (h) Serum prolactin

3   A 35-year-old woman was admitted with a manic episode with psychotic features. She has been treated with intramuscular haloperidol for the past 3 days because of high levels of agitation and refusal to adhere with oral medication. She presents with a temperature of 38.5 °C, confusion and muscle rigidity.
   (f) Creatine kinase

Treatment interventions

Options:

- (a) Start aripiprazole
- (b) Start metformin
- (c) Diet and exercise plan
- (d) Start atorvastatin
- (e) Stop clozapine
- (f) Start depot medication
- (g) Start antidepressant medication
- (h) Start methylphenidate

Select two interventions from the options above that would be recommended for each of the following clinical scenarios.

1 A 30-year-old man with a diagnosis of schizophrenia has remained stable while treated with olanzapine for the past 5 years. At his 6-monthly physical health check-up, he presents with two consecutive fasting serum glucose levels of 7.5 mmol/L (reference range 0–6.9 mmol/L) and has a HbA1c of 6.9% (52 mmol/mol) (reference range 4.0–5.9% (20–41 mmol/mol)).

(b) Start metformin
(c) Diet and exercise plan

2 A 32-year-old woman has been treated for the past 3 months with clozapine. She presents with weight gain. She has recently completed a diet and exercise programme but without any improvement in her weight.

(a) Start aripiprazole
(b) Start metformin ?

3 A 36-year-old woman with schizophrenia has been stable while treated with clozapine for the past 10 years. At her 6-monthly physical health check-up, she has elevated serum cholesterol at 6.7 mmol/L (reference range 0–5.0 mmol/L) and an elevated low-density-lipoprotein cholesterol, at 4.1 mmol/L (reference range 0–3.0 mmol/L). This is the second occasion that she has had similar abnormal blood results.

(c) Diet and exercise plan
(d) Start atorvastatin

CHAPTER 9

Pharmacological treatments

MCQs

1 Which of the following antipsychotic agents is least likely to be associated with weight gain?

   (a)   Olanzapine
   (b)   Clozapine
   (c)   Aripiprazole
   (d)   Risperidone
   (e)   Quetiapine

2 Which of the following is the least likely side-effect of tricyclic antidepressants?

   (a)   Sedation
   (b)   Urinary retention
   (c)   Blurred vision
   (d)   Dizziness
   (e)   Diarrhoea

3 A 22-year-old man started on a typical antipsychotic finds it difficult to sit still and has to move his legs constantly. How is this phenomenon best defined?

   (a)   Tardive dyskinesia
   (b)   Akinesia
   (c)   Akathisia
   (d)   Neuroleptic malignant syndrome
   (e)   Acute dystonic reaction

4   A 28-year-old woman with a 5-year history of bipolar affective disorder, currently in remission, attends the out-patient clinic to discuss suitable medications that she could use during pregnancy. Which of the following medications would be the least safe to prescribe to a woman who is planning a pregnancy?

(a)   Fluoxetine
(b)   Sodium valproate
(c)   Chlorpromazine
(d)   Olanzapine
(e)   Lamotrigine

5   A 40-year-old man with treatment-resistant schizophrenia was recently started on a typical antipsychotic. He presents 7 days later with fever, motor rigidity, confusion and diaphoresis. The most likely diagnosis is:

(a)   Neuroleptic malignant syndrome
(b)   Acute renal failure
(c)   Hyponatraemia
(d)   Tardive dyskinesia
(e)   Akathisia

6   Which of the following has the most clearly defined therapeutic range?

(a)   Paliperidone
(b)   Nortriptyline
(c)   Lithium carbonate
(d)   Quetiapine
(e)   Lamotrigine

7   Which of the following symptoms is related to lithium toxicity?

(a)   Polydipsia
(b)   Polyuria
(c)   Metallic taste
(d)   Coarse tremor
(e)   Hypothyroidism

8   High plasma levels of clozapine lead to an increased risk of which of the following?

(a)   Headaches
(b)   Myocardial infarction
(c)   Rash
(d)   Seizures
(e)   Panic attacks

9   The CATIE and CUtLASS studies focused on what type of medications?

(a)   Antidepressants
(b)   Antipsychotics
(c)   Antiepileptics
(d)   Benzodiazepines
(e)   Chemotherapy agents

10 Which of the following is not a common adverse event that needs to be considered before choosing an antipsychotic drug?

(a)   Metabolic syndrome
(b)   Weight gain
(c)   Akathisia
(d)   Sedation
(e)   Gallstones

11 A patient who was recently started on a new antipsychotic medication has returned to the clinic reporting a tremor. Which of the following receptors is likely to be involved?

(a)   Serotonergic
(b)   Dopaminergic
(c)   Histaminergic
(d)   Alpha 2
(e)   Muscarinic

12 Which of the following medications is a prophylactic treatment used in alcohol dependence syndrome?

(a)   Disulfiram
(b)   Chlordiazepoxide
(c)   Diazepam
(d)   Fluoxetine
(e)   Bupropion

13 Antipsychotic medications are associated with all the following except:

(a)   Impaired glucose tolerance
(b)   Dyslipidaemia
(c)   Shortened QTc interval
(d)   Increased risk of cerebrovascular accidents
(e)   Amenorrhoea

14 A 60-year-old woman attends the out-patient clinic reporting feeling dizzy when she gets up in the morning and when standing from a sitting position. She has been treated with sertraline for a depressive illness and was recently started on quetiapine for the symptomatic treatment of anxiety. Which of the following is the most likely cause of her symptoms?

(a) Dehydration secondary to decreased appetite
(b) Serotonergic stimulation
(c) Hypoglycaemia
(d) Anticholinergic receptor antagonism
(e) Alpha-1-adrenergic receptor antagonism

15 Which is the most appropriate treatment for a 60-year-old man who presents with visual hallucinations, agitation and severe tremor in the context of alcohol withdrawal syndrome?

(a) Chlordiazepoxide
(b) Olanzapine
(c) Phenytoin
(d) Temazepam
(e) Haloperidol

16 A 40-year-old man with a diagnosis of bipolar affective disorder, currently in remission for 8 years on maintenance therapy with lithium carbonate, presents to the emergency department with features of lithium toxicity. Which of the following is most likely to have precipitated such a presentation?

(a) Clozapine
(b) Olanzapine
(c) Diclofenac
(d) Amiloride
(e) Amlodipine

17 A 40-year-old man with a 15-year history of paranoid schizophrenia attends the clinic and reports the recent re-emergence of auditory hallucinations. He had been stable while treated with clozapine and amisulpride. You learn that he has recently begun smoking after a 5-year period of abstinence. Which of the following would you expect to see?

(a) Decreased amisulpride levels
(b) Increased clozapine levels
(c) Decreased amisulpride and clozapine levels
(d) Decreased clozapine levels
(e) Increased amisulpride levels

18 Which of the following is an indication for use of a long-acting injectable (depot) antipsychotic?

    (a)   Preference expressed by patient
    (b)   Patient not responsive to two oral antipsychotics
    (c)   Convenience for a busy community psychiatric team
    (d)   Patient poorly tolerates first-generation antipsychotics
    (e)   Sedation and metabolic syndrome are problems

19 Gastrointestinal upset is a common early side-effect when using SSRIs. Which mechanism of receptor action is most responsible for this effect?

    (a) 5-HT_1 stimulation
    (b) 5-HT_3 stimulation
    (c) 5-HT_2 blockade
    (d) 5-HT_3 blockade
    (e) 5-HT_2 stimulation

20 Which of the following effects is mediated by the D2 receptor activity of antipsychotics?

    (a)   Sedation
    (b)   Hyperprolactinaemia
    (c)   Weight gain
    (d)   Postural hypotension
    (e)   Anti-emetic effect

21 A 25-year-old man with a diagnosis of paranoid schizophrenia has experienced a psychotic relapse. He is hospitalised and started on a new antipsychotic medication. Which of the following adverse events associated with antipsychotics is thought to increase the risk of suicide?

    (a)   Akathisia
    (b)   Neuroleptic malignant syndrome
    (c)   Dystonia
    (d)   Sedation
    (e)   Tremor

22 A 25-year-old man with a history of rapid-cycling bipolar affective disorder has recently started taking lamotrigine, in combination with his maintenance mood stabiliser, for the treatment of a depressive episode. He is commenced at a normal titration rate of lamotrigine but presents to the clinic with evidence of lamotrigine toxicity. Which of the following medications would be associated with increased serum lamotrigine levels?

    (a)   Carbamazepine
    (b)   Lithium carbonate
    (c)   Sodium valproate
    (d)   Olanzapine
    (e)   Haloperidol

23 A 30-year-old man with a history of paranoid schizophrenia has recently had bowel resection surgery for a gastrointestinal condition. Which of the following antipsychotics would be best prescribed in order to avoid absorption problems due to the bowel resection?

(a) Amisulpride
(b) Aripiprazole
(c) Clozapine
(d) Quetiapine
(e) Risperidone

24 Regarding combinations of antipsychotics, which of the following is true?

(a) There is little evidence to show potential for harm
(b) Combined antipsychotics are rarely prescribed in practice
(c) It is best to use two drugs in the same class
(d) There is very little evidence to support the efficacy of combined antipsychotics
(e) The combination of risperidone and aripiprazole has been shown to be effective

25 A 22-year-old woman is admitted to hospital following the ingestion of 40 tablets of unknown origin. Her physical examination is normal but she is admitted for serial observations. Approximately 30h after her overdose, she is found to have an aspartate aminotransferase (AST) level of 2000 IU/L (reference range 6–34 IU/L) and an alanine aminotransferase (ALT) level of 2500 IU/L (reference range 5–38 IU/L). What medication has she probably ingested?

(a) Ibuprofen
(b) Paracetamol
(c) Citalopram
(d) Prednisolone
(e) Aspirin

26 Which of the following is true regarding the negative symptoms of schizophrenia and their treatment?

(a) Haloperidol has a clear benefit over second-generation antipsychotics in treating negative symptoms
(b) Secondary negative symptoms might be due to medication side-effects
(c) Treatment with SSRIs is standard practice
(d) Patients who misuse psychoactive substances have more negative symptoms
(e) Negative symptoms are not a concern for clinicians

27 A 55-year-old woman attends the out-patient clinic with a number of symptoms that have proven resistant to multiple antidepressants. She has also been treated with diazepam for the past 5 years. All the following are side-effects associated with benzodiazepine use, except:

(a) Rebound insomnia
(b) Depression
(c) Anterograde amnesia
(d) Respiratory stimulation
(e) Confusion

28 A 26-year-old man was started on clozapine for treatment-resistant schizophrenia 2 weeks ago. At an out-patient clinic review, he was found to have a temperature of 38 °C, but his physical examination was otherwise normal. What would be the most appropriate action?

(a) Admit to hospital
(b) Prescribe an antibiotic
(c) Request a full blood count
(d) Request a creatine kinase test
(e) Start aripiprazole

EMI questions

Classification of psychotropic drugs

Options:

(a) SSRIs
(b) Atypical antipsychotics
(c) SNRIs
(d) Reversible monoamine oxidase inhibitors
(e) First-generation antipsychotics
(f) Mood stabilisers
(g) Noradrenaline–dopamine reuptake inhibitors
(h) Tricyclic antidepressants

The following agents are examples of which of the above groups of drugs? (Each option is used once only.)

1 Venlafaxine

2 Sodium valproate

3 Clomipramine

4 Bupropion

Adverse effects of antidepressants

Options:

(a) Sertraline
(b) Agomelatine
(c) Citalopram
(d) Amitriptyline
(e) Fluoxetine
(f) Moclobemide
(g) Venlafaxine (extended release)
(h) Paroxetine

For each of the vignettes below, please select the antidepressant that is most likely to have caused the adverse effect. (Each option may be used for more than one answer.)

1   A 24-year-old woman was prescribed an antidepressant 2 weeks ago. She self-discontinued the medication because of side-effects and returned to the out-patient clinic complaining of heightened anxiety, insomnia, dizziness and flu-like symptoms. These symptoms began within 2 days of stopping the antidepressant.

2   A 40-year-old man was recently started on an antidepressant medication by his GP. He showed little response to the treatment and was referred to the out-patient clinic after his GP discovered that his liver function was abnormal. Which of the above antidepressants specifically requires the monitoring of liver function in the first months of treatment?

3   A 32-year-old businessman attends your clinic and you diagnose him with a severe depressive episode. On mental state examination, suicidal ideation is identified. Which of the above antidepressants is associated with the greatest risk in such a clinical scenario?

4   A 50-year-old mother of two presents to your clinic 2 weeks after an increase in her antidepressant dose was prescribed because of residual symptoms of depression. She is reporting excess sedation. Which of the above antidepressants is most associated with sedation?

Monitoring for adverse events with psychotropic medications

Options:

(a) Full blood count
(b) Urea and electrolytes
(c) Thyroid function tests
(d) Plasma levels of the medication
(e) Liver function tests
(f) Annual fasting glucose and lipid profile
(g) Electrocardiogram

Select an investigation that is part of the standard monitoring procedure for the clinical scenarios described below. (There is more than one answer for each scenario and answers may be used more than once.)

1 A 23-year-old woman with treatment-resistant schizophrenia being treated with clozapine. (Select three options.)

2 A 45-year-old man with bipolar affective disorder on long-term lithium therapy. (Select three options.)

3 A 30-year-old man with schizoaffective disorder on olanzapine and citalopram. (Select two options.)

MCQ answers

1 Which of the following antipsychotic agents is least likely to be associated with weight gain?

(a) Olanzapine
(b) Clozapine
(c) **Aripiprazole**
(d) Risperidone
(e) Quetiapine

Aripiprazole has one of the most favourable side-effect profiles of all antipsychotic drugs, with relatively little incidence of weight gain, sedation, hyperprolactinaemia or anticholinergic side-effects.

One of the problematic side-effects of antipsychotic medication is the high prevalence of weight gain in this population. Antipsychotic drugs can have a considerable impact on weight. Of the second-generation antipsychotic drugs, clozapine and olanzapine cause the most weight gain, followed by risperidone and quetiapine. Less weight gain seems to be associated with aripiprazole and amisulpride. Treatment for weight gain consists mostly of lifestyle interventions. Another option is switching to a drug with lower weight gain capacity, such as aripiprazole. Aripiprazole treatment over 12 months is a significant predictor for weight loss and adding aripiprazole to clozapine is an option for overweight patients on clozapine. See Schorr *et al* (2008) and Taylor *et al* (2012).

2   Which of the following is the least likely side-effect of tricyclic antidepressants?
   (a)   Sedation
   (b)   Urinary retention
   (c)   Blurred vision
   (d)   Dizziness
   (e)   **Diarrhoea**

Common side-effects of tricyclic antidepressants include dry mouth, blurred vision, drowsiness, weight gain, constipation and cognitive impairment (especially in elderly patients). See Taylor *et al* (2012).

3   A 22-year-old man started on a typical antipsychotic finds it difficult to sit still and has to move his legs constantly. How is this phenomenon best defined?
   (a)   Tardive dyskinesia
   (b)   Akinesia
   (c)   **Akathisia**
   (d)   Neuroleptic malignant syndrome
   (e)   Acute dystonic reaction

The diagnosis and assessment of akathisia should take account of both its subjective and objective components. Commonly experienced subjective components are a sense of inner restlessness, mental unease, unrest or dysphoria, feeling unable to keep still, an irresistible urge to move the legs and mounting inner tension when required to stand still. Akathisia is considered a relatively common acute extrapyramidal problem, but it can also be a persistent problem in those receiving maintenance antipsychotic treatment. Several rating scales are available for the assessment of akathisia, of which the Barnes scale is the most widely used. See Gervin & Barnes (2000).

4   A 28-year-old woman with a 5-year history of bipolar affective disorder, currently in remission, attends the out-patient clinic to discuss suitable medications that she could use during pregnancy. Which of the following medications would be the least safe to prescribe to a woman who is planning a pregnancy?
   (a)   Fluoxetine
   (b)   **Sodium valproate**
   (c)   Chlorpromazine
   (d)   Olanzapine
   (e)   Lamotrigine

All psychotropic drugs carry some degree of risk when used in pregnancy and require careful consideration and open discussion with patients. Sodium valproate has a clear causal link with foetal abnormalities, particularly spina bifida, and should be avoided if possible in pregnancy.

SSRIs seem not to be major teratogens, with sertraline and fluoxetine best supported by data. Olanzapine seems to be safe in terms of congenital malformations but is associated with other problems, including neural tube defects and macroplasia. The risks associated with first-generation antipsychotics such as chlorpromazine seem to be relatively small. Lamotrigine has been associated with cleft palate but a relatively low risk of neural tube malformations, compared with sodium valproate. See James *et al* (2007), Taylor *et al* (2012) and Tomson *et al* (2015).

5   A 40-year-old man with treatment-resistant schizophrenia was recently started on a typical antipsychotic. He presents 7 days later with fever, motor rigidity, confusion and diaphoresis. The most likely diagnosis is:

    (a)   **Neuroleptic malignant syndrome**
    (b)   Acute renal failure
    (c)   Hyponatraemia
    (d)   Tardive dyskinesia
    (e)   Akathisia

Neuroleptic malignant syndrome is a rare but potentially lethal form of drug-induced hyperthermia characterised by mental status changes, muscle rigidity, hyperthermia and autonomic dysfunction. In early studies, the mortality rates were in the range 20–38%; however, in the past two decades mortality rates have fallen below 10% because of early recognition and improved management.

However, the diagnosis of neuroleptic malignant syndrome presents a challenge because several medical conditions generate similar symptoms, including serotonin syndrome. A recent international expert group study agreed on the following criteria:

▶ recent dopamine antagonist exposure or dopamine agonist withdrawal
▶ hyperthermia
▶ rigidity
▶ mental status alteration
▶ creatine kinase elevation
▶ sympathetic nervous system lability
▶ tachycardia plus tachypnoea
▶ negative work-up for other causes.

See Ahuja & Cole (2009), Gurrera *et al* (2011) and Velamoor (1998).

6   Which of the following has the most clearly defined therapeutic range?

    (a)   Paliperidone
    (b)   Nortriptyline
    (c)   **Lithium carbonate**
    (d)   Quetiapine
    (e)   Lamotrigine

Lithium has been used for decades as a mood stabiliser and its therapeutic range is clearly established, although guidelines differ slightly in the exact figures. The Maudsley Guidelines recommend a level of 0.6–1.0 mmol/L, which might be slightly higher in mania. Target ranges for quetiapine and lamotrigine are not clearly established. Target ranges for tricyclic antidepressants such as nortriptyline are rarely used and of questionable benefit. Paliperidone is a relatively new drug and limited data exist. See Schou (1997) and Taylor *et al* (2012).

7   Which of the following symptoms is related to lithium toxicity?

   (a)   Polydipsia
   (b)   Polyuria
   (c)   Metallic taste
   (d)   **Coarse tremor**
   (e)   Hypothyroidism

Coarse tremor is a sign of central nervous system toxicity. Polydipisia, polyuria, fine tremor and metallic taste are common adverse effects of lithium often seen in the early stages of treatment, whereas hypothyroidism is a common long-term side-effect, particularly in middle-aged women; however, none of these are typically related to toxicity. See Taylor *et al* (2012).

8   High plasma levels of clozapine lead to an increased risk of which of the following?

   (a)   Headaches
   (b)   Myocardial infarction
   (c)   Rash
   (d)   **Seizures**
   (e)   Panic attacks

Seizures occur more frequently in patients who receive doses > 500 mg/day and plasma levels above 600 ug/L. At this dose and level, prophylactic treatment with sodium valproate should be considered. See Taylor *et al* (2012) and Varma *et al* (2011).

9   The CATIE and CUtLASS studies focused on what type of medications?

   (a)   Antidepressants
   (b)   **Antipsychotics**
   (c)   Antiepileptics
   (d)   Benzodiazepines
   (e)   Chemotherapy agents

The CATIE and CUtLASS trials, published in 2005 and 2006, respectively, prompted an important rethink about the efficacy of second-generation antipsychotics. They called into question the common perception at the time that these drugs were far superior to their first-generation counterparts. In fact, these studies concluded that if extrapyramidal side-effects from first-generation agents could be minimised and anticholinergic use avoided, there was no convincing evidence to suggest the superiority of second-generation antipsychotics (with the exception of olanzapine and clozapine). See Jones *et al* (2006) and Lieberman *et al* (2005).

10 Which of the following is not a common adverse event that needs to be considered before choosing an antipsychotic drug?

(a) Metabolic syndrome
(b) Weight gain
(c) Akathisia
(d) Sedation
(e) **Gallstones**

Gallstones are not a common side-effect of any antipsychotic drug. The other answers are adverse events common to many antipsychotic drugs. Before choosing an antipsychotic drug, careful consideration should be given to the side-effect profile and the choice should be made in collaboration with the patient. Certain side-effects can be relatively more or less acceptable to different patients. See NICE (2014).

11 A patient who was recently started on a new antipsychotic medication has returned to the clinic reporting a tremor. Which of the following receptors is likely to be involved?

(a) Serotonergic
(b) **Dopaminergic**
(c) Histaminergic
(d) Alpha 2
(e) Muscarinic

Striatal D2 occupancy predicts antipsychotic response, but also drug-induced extrapyramidal side-effects, akathisia, and prolactin elevation. There is evidence for a stepped increase in clinical response beyond 65% D2 occupancy. However, at >72% D2 occupancy, side-effects relating to D2 blockade are more likely. Prolactin elevation has been shown to be prominent beyond 72%, while extra-pyramidal side-effects and akathisia are evident beyond 78%.

The optimal treatment strategy is to achieve the highest rate of response with the lowest incidence of side-effects. Therefore, the therapeutic window for antipsychotics has been postulated to be between 65% and 72% D2 occupancy. Compared with first-generation (typical) antipsychotics, second-generation (atypical) antipsychotics have a lower liability for extrapyramidal side-effects. See Gervin & Barnes (2000) and Kapur *et al* (2000).

12 Which of the following medications is a prophylactic treatment used in alcohol dependence syndrome?

(a) **Disulfiram**
(b) Chlordiazepoxide
(c) Diazepam
(d) Fluoxetine
(e) Bupropion

Disulfiram is an inhibitor of hepatic aldehyde dehydrogenase and blocks the oxidation of alcohol, causing an accumulation of acetaldehyde after drinking.

This leads to a very unpleasant and potentially dangerous physiological state. Recent guidelines suggest disulfiram should be considered as a prophylactic treatment, in combination with a psychological intervention, in patients with moderate to severe alcohol dependence who want to achieve abstinence but for whom acamprosate and oral naltrexone are not suitable, or in patients who prefer disulfiram and understand the risks involved. See Fuller & Gordis (2004) and NICE (2011*a*).

13 Antipsychotic medications are associated with all the following except:
- (a) Impaired glucose tolerance
- (b) Dyslipidaemia
- (c) **Shortened QTc interval**
- (d) Increased risk of cerebrovascular accidents
- (e) Amenorrhoea

The QTc interval remains the most valid surrogate marker for torsades de pointes, and prolongation to > 500 ms is associated with an increased risk of torsades de pointes. From the point of view of cardiac safety, antipsychotics should be used in monotherapy at recommended dosages and not in combination with other drugs prolonging the QTc interval. Special precautions, such as performing an electrocardiogram and monitoring serum electrolyte levels (specifically serum potassium and magnesium levels where there are clinical concerns), should always be observed. The antipsychotics thioridazine, sertindole and ziprasidone have all been associated with severe QTc prolongation. See Nielsen *et al* (2011).

14 A 60-year-old woman attends the out-patient clinic reporting feeling dizzy when she gets up in the morning and when standing from a sitting position. She has been treated with sertraline for a depressive illness and was recently started on quetiapine for the symptomatic treatment of anxiety. Which of the following is the most likely cause of her symptoms?
- (a) Dehydration secondary to decreased appetite
- (b) Serotonergic stimulation
- (c) Hypoglycaemia
- (d) Anticholinergic receptor antagonism
- (e) **Alpha-1-adrenergic receptor antagonism**

Alpha-1-adrenergic antagonism (i.e. receptor blockade) can cause postural hypotension and dizziness, potentiation of the antihypertensive effect of other medications, reflex tachycardia and sexual dysfunction (orgasmic failure/delay in men). Antipsychotics with a pronounced alpha-1-adrenergic effect include clozapine, risperidone and quetiapine. These agents must be gradually titrated to therapeutic dosing, in order to avoid the occurrence of side-effects such as postural hypotension. See Taylor *et al* (2012).

15 Which is the most appropriate treatment for a 60-year-old man who presents with visual hallucinations, agitation and severe tremor in the context of alcohol withdrawal syndrome?

   (a)   **Chlordiazepoxide**
   (b)   Olanzapine
   (c)   Phenytoin
   (d)   Temazepam
   (e)   Haloperidol

Acute alcohol withdrawal syndrome encompasses the physical and psychological symptoms that people can experience when they suddenly reduce the amount of alcohol they drink, if they have previously been drinking excessively for prolonged periods of time. Medically assisted alcohol withdrawal requires benzodiazepines as first-line treatment to control symptoms. Chlordiazepoxide and diazepam are the two most commonly used benzodiazepines for this indication. For people in acute alcohol withdrawal who have developed, or are assessed to be at high risk of developing, alcohol withdrawal seizures or delirium tremens, hospital admission for medically assisted alcohol withdrawal should be offered. See NICE (2010).

16 A 40-year-old man with a diagnosis of bipolar affective disorder, currently in remission for 8 years on maintenance therapy with lithium carbonate, presents to the emergency department with features of lithium toxicity. Which of the following is most likely to have precipitated such a presentation?

   (a)   Clozapine
   (b)   Olanzapine
   (c)   **Diclofenac**
   (d)   Amiloride
   (e)   Amlodipine

Lithium is dangerous in overdose or in circumstances that predispose to sodium or volume depletion. Most patients who experience lithium toxicity do so when they are ill (diarrhoea, vomiting, heart failure, renal failure, or surgery) or secondary to a drug interaction, such as non-steroidal anti-inflammatory drugs (NSAIDs) or angiotensin-converting-enzyme inhibitors. NSAIDs such as diclofenac can increase the reabsorption of lithium by the kidney and result in increased serum lithium concentrations.

Clinical signs of toxicity usual emerge at concentrations of 1.5 mmol/L or greater. The present guidance, to monitor serum lithium concentrations every 3 months, is mainly aimed at avoiding drift into the toxic range (as well as ensuring that therapeutic levels are maintained), but evidence to support this approach is scarce. See McKnight *et al* (2012).

17 A 40-year-old man with a 15-year history of paranoid schizophrenia attends the clinic and reports the recent re-emergence of auditory hallucinations. He had been stable while treated with clozapine and amisulpride. You learn that he has recently begun smoking after a 5-year period of abstinence. Which of the following would you expect to see?

(a) Decreased amisulpride levels
(b) Increased clozapine levels
(c) Decreased amisulpride and clozapine levels
(d) **Decreased clozapine levels**
(e) Increased amisulpride levels

Smoking has a large effect on clozapine metabolism. Smoking can induce hepatic cytochrome P450 (CYP) oxidative enzymes, in particular CYP1A2, thus reducing serum levels of medications metabolised by these enzymes. Nicotine itself does not seem to exert important effects on the CYP drug metabolizing system, but polycyclic hydrocarbons in cigarette smoke can induce some microsomal oxidases, including the CYP1A2 isoform, which is implicated as part of the metabolism of clozapine. Smokers with schizophrenia therefore require higher doses of clozapine. Amisulpride is not extensively hepatically metabolised. See Cormac *et al* (2010) and Derenne & Baldessarini (2005).

18 Which of the following is an indication for use of a long-acting injectable (depot) antipsychotic?

(a) **Preference expressed by patient**
(b) Patient not responsive to two oral antipsychotics
(c) Convenience for a busy community psychiatric team
(d) Patient poorly tolerates first-generation antipsychotics
(e) Sedation and metabolic syndrome are problems

Long-acting injections (depots) are recommended where a patient has expressed a preference for it and where avoiding covert non-adherence is a priority. Convenience in general is a consideration, but not just the team's convenience – the patient should be agreeable whenever possible. Depot formulations are available for both first-generation and second-generation antipsychotics, so drug choice should be tailored to tolerability (as with oral medication). A patient not being responsive to two oral antipsychotic agents (assuming adherence and adequate trial) is an indication for treatment with clozapine, not depots. See NICE (2014).

19 Gastrointestinal upset is a common early side-effect when using SSRIs. Which mechanism of receptor action is most responsible for this effect?

(a) 5-HT_1 stimulation
(b) **5-HT_3 stimulation**
(c) 5-HT_2 blockade
(d) 5-HT_3 blockade
(e) 5-HT_2 stimulation

SSRI side-effects can be predicted from their receptor physiology. Most side-effects are dose-related and can be attributed to serotonergic effects. The improved tolerability of the SSRIs (compared with older antidepressants) is due to their selectivity and the fact they do not interact with other receptors, such as histaminic, cholinergic, dopaminergic and noradrenergic receptors.

Gastrointestinal side-effects are most commonly reported. They probably result from stimulation of 5-HT$_3$ receptors. Nausea and diarrhoea usually resolve within the first 2 weeks of treatment. They are dose-related and can usually be alleviated by reducing the SSRI dose. Starting the medication at a low dose and giving it with food often alleviates nausea. Fluvoxamine and sertraline the SSRIs most commonly associated with gastrointestinal side-effects. See Ferguson (2001) and Goldstein & Goodnick (1998).

20 Which of the following effects is mediated by the D2 receptor activity of antipsychotics?

    (a)   Sedation
    (b)   **Hyperprolactinaemia**
    (c)   Weight gain
    (d)   Postural hypotension
    (e)   Anti-emetic effect

Dopamine is the predominant prolactin-inhibiting factor in humans. Blockade of D2 receptors removes the primary inhibiting factor of prolactin secretion, thereby stimulating anterior pituitary lactotroph proliferation and prolactin secretion. Symptoms of hyperprolactinaemia include gynaecomastia, galactorrhoea, sexual dysfunction, infertility, oligomenorrhoea and amenorrhoea. All D2 antagonists can trigger hyperprolactinaemia but it is most commonly associated with amisulpride, risperidone, haloperidol and other first-generation antipsychotics. See Bushe *et al* (2008) and Haddad & Wieck (2004).

21 A 25-year-old man with a diagnosis of paranoid schizophrenia has experienced a psychotic relapse. He is hospitalised and started on a new antipsychotic medication. Which of the following adverse events associated with antipsychotics is thought to increase the risk of suicide?

    (a)   **Akathisia**
    (b)   Neuroleptic malignant syndrome
    (c)   Dystonia
    (d)   Sedation
    (e)   Tremor

It has been suggested that akathisia often exacerbates psychotic agitation and that the diagnosis should be considered whenever a patient develops impulsive suicidal ideation after a change in neuroleptic treatment.

However, in a critical review of the literature, akathisia was not unequivocally linked to suicidal behaviour. The authors noted that the condition causes considerable distress in an already vulnerable group of patients and recommended that new, more rigorous strategies be put in place to prevent it. See Drake & Ehrlich (1985) and Hansen (2001).

22 A 25-year-old man with a history of rapid-cycling bipolar affective disorder has recently started taking lamotrigine, in combination with his maintenance mood stabiliser, for the treatment of a depressive episode. He is commenced at a normal titration rate of lamotrigine but presents to the clinic with evidence of lamotrigine toxicity. Which of the following medications would be associated with increased serum lamotrigine levels?

    (a)   Carbamazepine
    (b)   Lithium carbonate
    (c)   **Sodium valproate**
    (d)   Olanzapine
    (e)   Haloperidol

Sodium valproate is a widely used anticonvulsant drug with a broad therapeutic spectrum. It is an inhibitor of cytochrome P450 liver enzymes and in this way causes reduced elimination (and hence potentially increased levels) of drugs metabolised by these enzymes, such as lamotrigine. See Choi & Morrell (2003) and Gunes *et al* (2007).

23 A 30-year-old man with a history of paranoid schizophrenia has recently had bowel resection surgery for a gastrointestinal condition. Which of the following antipsychotics would be best prescribed in order to avoid absorption problems due to the bowel resection?

    (a)   Amisulpride
    (b)   Aripiprazole
    (c)   Clozapine
    (d)   Quetiapine
    (e)   **Risperidone**

This question requires some lateral thinking! As this man has had a bowel resection, injectable depot medication is preferable. Of the answers given, only risperidone is available in depot form. See Taylor *et al* (2012).

24 Regarding combinations of antipsychotics, which of the following is true?

    (a)   There is little evidence to show potential for harm
    (b)   Combined antipsychotics are rarely prescribed in practice
    (c)   It is best to use two drugs in the same class
    (d)   **There is very little evidence to support the efficacy of combined antipsychotics**
    (e)   The combination of risperidone and aripiprazole has been shown to be effective

There is very little evidence to support the efficacy of combined antipsychotics, and substantial evidence supports the potential for harm. Despite this, the practice is widespread and seems difficult to change. If a combination is deemed absolutely necessary, a rational, evidence-based approach is recommended. There is some evidence for clozapine augmentation strategies and for the use of aripiprazole to reduce weight in those on clozapine and reduce hyperprolactinaemia in those on haloperidol. See Barbui *et al* (2009), Kane *et al* (2009) and Taylor *et al* (2012).

25 A 22-year-old woman is admitted to hospital following the ingestion of 40 tablets of unknown origin. Her physical examination is normal but she is admitted for serial observations. Approximately 30 h after her overdose, she is found to have an aspartate aminotransferase (AST) level of 2000 IU/L (reference range 6–34 IU/L) and an alanine aminotransferase (ALT) level of 2500 IU/L (reference range 5–38 IU/L). What medication has she probably ingested?

    (a)   Ibuprofen
    (b)   **Paracetamol**
    (c)   Citalopram
    (d)   Prednisolone
    (e)   Aspirin

Paracetamol leads to delayed liver damage because its standard metabolism by glucuronidation is quickly saturated by an overdose. Production of the toxic metabolite of paracetamol, N-acetyl-p-benzoquinone imine, in excess of an adequate store of conjugating glutathione, is associated with hepatocellular damage, necrosis and hepatic failure.

Toxicity is associated with a single acute paracetamol ingestion of 150 mg/kg or approximately 7–10 g in adults. A serum paracetamol concentration drawn ≥ 4 h after a single ingestion should be plotted on the Rumack–Matthew nomogram as a guide to predicting the likelihood of potential hepatotoxicity and need for N-acetylcysteine therapy. AST and ALT levels begin to rise within 24 h of acute ingestion and peak at about 72 h. See Whyte *et al* (2007).

26 Which of the following is true regarding the negative symptoms of schizophrenia and their treatment?

    (a)   Haloperidol has a clear benefit over second-generation antipsychotics in treating negative symptoms
    (b)   **Secondary negative symptoms might be due to medication side-effects**
    (c)   Treatment with SSRIs is standard practice
    (d)   Patients who misuse psychoactive substances have more negative symptoms
    (e)   Negative symptoms are not a concern for clinicians

Negative symptoms of schizophrenia can be severely debilitating for patients and warrant significant attention from clinicians. Negative symptoms can be primary (due to schizophrenia itself), or secondary to positive symptoms, depression, institutionalisation or drug side-effects (sedation and extra-pyramidal side-effects).

First-generation antipsychotics, such as haloperidol, have only a small effect on primary negative symptoms and can cause secondary negative symptoms via extra-pyramidal side-effects. Some second-generation antipsychotics have been shown to be more effective than first-generation antipsychotics in treating negative symptoms, but to date no single drug has shown a clear-cut benefit over the others. Other studies suggest a role for SSRIs, but this is not presently standard practice. Patients who use psychoactive substances have fewer negative symptoms, but it is not clear if this is a cause or an effect. See Leucht *et al* (2009) and Taylor *et al* (2012).

27 A 55-year-old woman attends the out-patient clinic with a number of symptoms that have proven resistant to multiple antidepressants. She has also been treated with diazepam for the past 5 years. All the following are side-effects associated with benzodiazepine use, except:

(a) Rebound insomnia
(b) Depression
(c) Anterograde amnesia
(d) **Respiratory stimulation**
(e) Confusion

Although uncommonly fatal in overdose, benzodiazepines can cause respiratory depression and hence can be dangerous when used in association with alcohol or other respiratory depressants. The most common side-effect of benzodiazepines is sedation. They can also cause psychomotor impairment and confusion in the elderly. On abrupt discontinuation of benzodiazepines after a sustained period of use, symptoms of anxiety, insomnia, amnesia, nausea, weakness, and hypersensitivity to light, sound, smell or taste can all occur. See Starcevic (2012).

28 A 26-year-old man was started on clozapine for treatment-resistant schizophrenia 2 weeks ago. At an out-patient clinic review, he was found to have a temperature of 38 °C, but his physical examination was otherwise normal. What would be the most appropriate action?

(a) Admit to hospital
(b) Prescribe an antibiotic
(c) **Request a full blood count**
(d) Request a creatine kinase test
(e) Start aripiprazole

A benign fever can occur in patients during the initial phase of clozapine treatment. This fever is not usually related to blood dyscrasias. However, a persistent rise in temperature raises concern about the possibility of agranulocytosis and infection. A full blood count with a white blood cell count and differential should be requested as a first-line investigation to rule out neutropenia. An antipyretic might be prescribed and consideration given to reducing the rate of dose titration. See Taylor *et al* (2012).

EMI answers

Classification of psychotropic drugs

Options:

- (a) SSRIs
- (b) Atypical antipsychotics
- (c) SNRIs
- (d) Reversible monoamine oxidase inhibitors
- (e) First-generation antipsychotics
- (f) Mood stabilisers
- (g) Noradrenaline–dopamine reuptake inhibitors
- (h) Tricyclic antidepressants

The following agents are examples of which of the above groups of drugs? (Each option is used once only.)

1 Venlafaxine
   (c) SNRIs

2 Sodium valproate
   (f) Mood stabilisers

3 Clomipramine
   (h) Tricyclic antidepressants

4 Bupropion
   (g) Noradrenaline–dopamine reuptake inhibitors

Adverse effects of antidepressants

Options:

- (a) Sertraline
- (b) Agomelatine
- (c) Citalopram
- (d) Amitriptyline
- (e) Fluoxetine
- (f) Moclobemide
- (g) Venlafaxine (extended release)
- (h) Paroxetine

For each of the vignettes below, please select the antidepressant that is most likely to have caused the adverse effect. (Each option may be used for more than one answer).

1 A 24-year-old woman was prescribed an antidepressant 2 weeks ago. She self-discontinued the medication because of side-effects and returned to the out-patient clinic complaining of heightened anxiety, insomnia, dizziness and flu-like symptoms. These symptoms began within 2 days of stopping the antidepressant.
   (h) Paroxetine

2   A 40-year-old man was recently started on an antidepressant medication by his GP.
He showed little response to the treatment and was referred to the out-patient clinic
after his GP discovered that his liver function was abnormal. Which of the above
antidepressants specifically requires the monitoring of liver function in the first
months of treatment?

(b) Agomelatine

3   A 32-year-old businessman attends your clinic and you diagnose him with a severe
depressive episode. On mental state examination, suicidal ideation is identified.
Which of the above antidepressants is associated with the greatest risk in such a
clinical scenario?

(d) Amitriptyline

4   A 50-year-old mother of two presents to your clinic 2 weeks after an increase in her
antidepressant dose was prescribed because of residual symptoms of depression. She
is reporting excess sedation. Which of the above antidepressants is most associated
with sedation?

(d) Amitriptyline

Monitoring for adverse events with psychotropic medications

Options:

(a)   Full blood count
(b)   Urea and electrolytes
(c)   Thyroid function tests
(d)   Plasma levels of the medication
(e)   Liver function tests
(f)   Annual fasting glucose and lipid profile
(g)   Electrocardiogram

Select an investigation that is part of the standard monitoring procedure for the clinical
scenarios described below. (There is more than one answer for each scenario and
answers may be used more than once.)

1   A 23-year-old woman with treatment-resistant schizophrenia being treated with
clozapine.

(a) Full blood count
(f) Annual fasting glucose and lipid profile
(g) Electrocardiogram

2   A 45-year-old man with bipolar affective disorder on long-term lithium therapy.

(b) Urea and electrolytes
(c) Thyroid function tests
(d) Plasma levels of the medication

3   A 30-year-old man with schizoaffective disorder on olanzapine and citalopram.

(f) Annual fasting glucose and lipid profile
(g) Electrocardiogram

CHAPTER 10

Psychology and psychotherapy

MCQs

1 Which psychiatrist introduced psychoanalysis?
   (a) Carl Jung
   (b) Sigmund Freud
   (c) Melanie Klein
   (d) Anna Freud
   (e) RD Laing

2 According to Freud, which part of the mind deals with primitive and instinctual impulses?
   (a) Subconscious
   (b) Ego
   (c) Id
   (d) Preconscious
   (e) Superego

3 Who described the terms 'introversion', 'extraversion' and 'archetypes'?
   (a) Sigmund Freud
   (b) Melanie Klein
   (c) Karl Popper
   (d) Carl Jung
   (e) John Bowlby

4 A 28-year-old man loses his job and moves back into his parents' house. While he is there, he does not tidy up after himself and begins to play computer games from his adolescence. What is the defence mechanism employed here?
   (a) Repression
   (b) Sublimation
   (c) Regression
   (d) Projection
   (e) Denial

5   A child beginning to walk cries when he stumbles and falls. His parents initially comfort him but over time stop doing this. He then learns to get up again when he stumbles. What is this is an example of?

(a)   Operant conditioning
(b)   Modelling
(c)   Attachment formation
(d)   Classical conditioning
(e)   Behavioural activation

6   The process in childhood by which clear-cut emotional bonds crucial to psychological development are made is called:

(a)   Bonding
(b)   Emotion formation
(c)   Parental guidance
(d)   Nurturing
(e)   Attachment

7   A 23-year-old man has had low mood for the past 2 months. He also describes reduced energy, insomnia and poor concentration. He feels hopeless about the future and he tells you that everything he does is a failure, despite having done well on his university exams. The psychological therapy that should be recommended for him is:

(a)   Psychoanalysis
(b)   Dialectical behaviour therapy
(c)   Cognitive–behavioural therapy
(d)   Cognitive analytical therapy
(e)   Group therapy

8   A 38-year-old woman reports feeling very anxious when she has to go to crowded places, particularly the supermarket. On one occasion, she experienced a panic attack. Which cognitive–behavioural therapy technique would be most useful in treating this patient?

(a)   Socratic questioning
(b)   Flooding
(c)   Systematic desensitisation
(d)   Addressing cognitive distortions
(e)   Homework exercises

9 A 19-year-old man says that he is 'scared to death' of spiders and cannot sleep at night, as he thinks there might be some in his room. When he last saw a spider, he became very frightened and felt he was going to faint. What psychological approach would be useful in treating this man?

(a) Psychoanalysis
(b) Exposure and response prevention
(c) Systematic desensitisation
(d) Addressing cognitive distortions
(e) Group therapy

10 A 21-year-old man becomes extremely distressed when his advances towards a woman in his university class are rejected. He feels it is very unfair that his feelings are not reciprocated as he cares deeply about her. He says that this always happens to him and that he has no hope of finding love in his life. He downplays the fact that two other women have expressed an interest in him. He believes that someone at his age should have a girlfriend. How would you categorise his thoughts in psychological terms?

(a) Immature thinking
(b) Extraversion
(c) Acting out
(d) Cognitive distortions
(e) Intellectualisation

11 A 37-year-old woman with a long-term history of depressive illness is referred to a psychologist for psychotherapy. The therapist encourages her to gain an understanding of the effect of her unconscious feelings on her relationships with her family. She also encourages her to make a connection between her past and present relationships. What type of therapy is being used here?

(a) Cognitive–behavioural therapy
(b) Interpersonal psychotherapy
(c) Cognitive analytical therapy
(d) Psychodynamic psychotherapy
(e) Schema therapy

12 A 21-year-old woman is preoccupied with her weight. She often binge-eats and subsequently causes herself to vomit. Her BMI is in the normal range. Which psychological treatments have been shown to be most effective for this condition?

(a) Psychoanalysis and cognitive–behavioural therapy (CBT)
(b) CBT and interpersonal psychotherapy
(c) Cognitive therapy and psychoanalysis
(d) Group therapy and supportive psychotherapy
(e) CBT and supportive psychotherapy

13 A 36-year-old man from Afghanistan describes intense 'reliving' of episodes of torture he experienced 10 years ago. He has nightmares about what happened to him and describes a heightened state of alert, especially at night while trying to sleep. He has begun to avoid public transport, as he was abducted while on a bus prior to his torture. What two types of psychological therapy are indicated for this man?

   (a) Trauma-focused cognitive–behavioural therapy (CBT) and eye movement desensitisation and reprocessing (EMDR)
   (b) Psychoanalysis and CBT
   (c) Debriefing and CBT
   (d) Interpersonal psychotherapy and EMDR
   (e) Supportive psychotherapy and psychoanalysis

EMI questions

Defence mechanisms

Options:
   (a) Splitting
   (b) Projection
   (c) Rationalisation
   (d) Regression
   (e) Repression
   (f) Reaction formation
   (g) Displacement
   (h) Dissociation

From the list above, choose the defence mechanism being used in each example below.

1 A 25-year-old woman who is struggling in her job because of her drinking habits tells herself that the problem is her difficult boss. She denies that her drinking has increased in frequency and severity and also blames the commute to work for her problems.

2 A 65-year-old man is frustrated with his physical health difficulties and decreasing ability to engage in social activities. He becomes more and more irritable with his wife, who cannot understand this change in him.

3 A 15-year-old boy with separated parents who has been disruptive at school becomes angry with his mother, saying she is evil and he never wants to speak to her again. On the other hand, he tells her his father is a great Dad and would never treat him this way.

Choice of psychotherapy

Options:

- (a) Cognitive–behavioural therapy
- (b) Cognitive analytical therapy
- (c) Dialectical behavioural therapy
- (d) Interpersonal psychotherapy
- (e) Psychodynamic psychotherapy
- (f) Psychoanalysis
- (g) Family therapy
- (h) Grief counselling

From the list above, choose the most appropriate choice of therapy for each of the examples below. More than one therapy may be used for each scenario.

1. A 19-year-old woman with bulimia nervosa.

2. A 22-year-old man demonstrating over-generalisation and somatisation.

3. A 45-year-old woman with long-term relationship difficulties and a history of conflict in her family.

4. A 65-year-old man having a prolonged grief reaction and symptoms of depression following the death of his wife.

5. A 26-year-old man with emotionally unstable personality disorder and repeated self-harm.

MCQ answers

1. Which psychiatrist introduced psychoanalysis?
   - (a) Carl Jung
   - (b) **Sigmund Freud**
   - (c) Melanie Klein
   - (d) Anna Freud
   - (e) RD Laing

Sigmund Freud was a key figure in the development of psychological therapy through his formation of the school of psychoanalysis. In his early work, he developed the concept of free association, which consisted of allowing his patients to speak in an undirected and non-judgemental way about their thoughts and feelings. In this way, he believed patients would access their unconscious mind and discover more about their true nature. He also developed the idea of transference, where patient's ideas and feelings about their past relationships are transferred to the therapist. Transference and counter-transference (feelings that the patient invokes in the therapist) remain important concepts in modern psychiatry and psychotherapy. See Cowen *et al* (2012) and, for further reading, Storr (2001).

2 According to Freud, which part of the mind deals with primitive and instinctual impulses?

   (a)   Subconscious
   (b)   Ego
   (c)   **Id**
   (d)   Preconscious
   (e)   Superego

Freud described two key models of mind – the topographical model and the structural model. The topographical model divides the mind into the conscious, preconscious and unconscious. He largely replaced this model with the structural model, which consists of the id, ego and superego. The id represents a human's basic instincts and drives, and operates only on the 'pleasure principle', seeking satisfaction without realism or foresight. The ego is concerned with mediating between the urgings of the id and the realities of the external world and operates on the 'reality principle'. The superego is concerned with self-observation, self-criticism and moral considerations. The ego and the superego are both viewed to be partly conscious and partly unconscious. See Martin *et al* (2013).

3 Who described the terms 'introversion', 'extraversion' and 'archetypes'?

   (a)   Sigmund Freud
   (b)   Melanie Klein
   (c)   Karl Popper
   (d)   **Carl Jung**
   (e)   John Bowlby

Carl Jung was an early follower of Freud who went on to develop his own psychological theories, drawing on religion, spirituality and philosophy. He agreed with Freud's model of the unconscious, but proposed the existence of a second, deeper form of the unconscious underlying this 'personal' one. He termed this the collective unconscious, which consisted of archetypes – hidden forms that are transformed once they enter consciousness and are given particular expression by individuals and their cultures. He also introduced the concepts of introversion (the state of or tendency towards being wholly or predominantly concerned with and interested in one's own mental life) and extraversion (the state of or tendency towards being predominantly concerned with and obtaining gratification from what is outside the self). See Stevens (2001) and, for further reading, Jung (1961).

4 A 28-year-old man loses his job and moves back into his parents' house. While he is there, he does not tidy up after himself and begins to play computer games from his adolescence. What is the defence mechanism employed here?

   (a)   Repression
   (b)   Sublimation
   (c)   **Regression**
   (d)   Projection
   (e)   Denial

Defence mechanisms refer to behaviours employed by individuals to cope with their own unacceptable thoughts and feelings. Defence mechanisms reduce anxiety by allowing the expression of the undesirable impulses or desires without becoming consciously aware of them. They can also be employed to allow the individual to cope with external stressors and frustrations. The term was introduced by Sigmund Freud but others such as Anna Freud, Otto Kernberg and George Valliant later expanded on the literature in this area. According to Valliant, defence mechanisms can be pathological (e.g. acting out, splitting), immature (e.g. idealisation), neurotic (e.g. displacement) or mature (e.g. humour, sublimation). Regression is an immature defence mechanism that involves temporary reversion to an earlier stage of psychological development. See Cowen *et al* (2012) and, for further reading, Cramer (2000).

5   A child beginning to walk cries when he stumbles and falls. His parents initially comfort him but over time stop doing this. He then learns to get up again when he stumbles. What is this is an example of?

(a)   **Operant conditioning**
(b)   Modelling
(c)   Attachment formation
(d)   Classical conditioning
(e)   Behavioural activation

Operant conditioning is a type of learning in which an individual's behaviour is modified by its antecedents and consequences. It forms the basis of behavioural psychology and behavioural therapy, as developed by Edward Thorndike and BF Skinner.

This differs from classical conditioning, which is based on stimuli that result in physiological effects. Pavlov's experiments with dogs were key to the understanding of classical conditioning. A conditioned stimulus (e.g. a bell rung when giving a dog food) is paired with an unconditioned stimulus (e.g. the food). The dog initially salivates because of the food (unconditioned response) but comes to associate the bell with food and so eventually salivates when it hears the bell (conditioned response). Although a more primitive form of learning, classical conditioning is used in behavioural therapy techniques such as aversion therapy, systematic desensitisation and flooding. See Martin *et al* (2013).

6   A 2-year-old child has formed a close connection with his mother. The process in childhood by which clear-cut emotional bonds crucial to psychological development are made is called:

(a)   Bonding
(b)   Emotion formation
(c)   Parental guidance
(d)   Nurturing
(e)   **Attachment**

Attachment theory was developed by John Bowlby. The theory is based on the idea that a child needs a secure relationship with at least one parent (or primary caregiver) in order to achieve emotional maturity. Insecure attachments lead to a range of emotional difficulties in later life, primarily in the formation of relationships. Insecure attachment is increasingly recognised as a risk factor for the development of personality disorders.

Pre-attachment behaviour occurs in the first 6 months of life. Clear-cut attachment develops in the third phase, between the ages of 6 months and 2 years. The infant's behaviour towards the caregiver becomes organised and goal-directed to achieve conditions that make them feel secure. After the second year, the child begins to see the caregiver as an independent person and a more complex partnership is formed. Cowen *et al* (2012) and, for further reading, Bowlby (1999) and Levy (2005).

7 A 23-year-old man has had low mood for the past 2 months. He also describes reduced energy, insomnia and poor concentration. He feels hopeless about the future and he tells you that everything he does is a failure, despite having done well on his university exams. The psychological therapy that should be recommended for him is:

   (a) Psychoanalysis
   (b) Dialectical behaviour therapy
   (c) **Cognitive–behavioural therapy**
   (d) Cognitive analytical therapy
   (e) Group therapy

Cognitive–behavioural therapy (CBT) is a psychological therapy that focuses on the interaction between thoughts, feelings and behaviour. It combines elements of cognitive therapy and behavioural therapy.

This man is having a moderate depressive episode with somatic features. He is also demonstrating cognitive distortions (magnification and minimisation), which are a focus of CBT. NICE guidelines for the treatment of moderate depressive episodes suggest the use of antidepressant medication in combination with CBT.

CBT has been proven to be effective in the treatment of mild and moderate depression. The evidence for its efficacy in severe depression is less conclusive. See Cowen *et al* (2012) and NICE (2009a) and, for further reading, Lynch *et al* (2010).

8 A 38-year-old woman reports feeling very anxious when she has to go to crowded places, particularly the supermarket. On one occasion, she experienced a panic attack. Which cognitive–behavioural therapy technique would be most useful in treating this patient?

   (a) Socratic questioning
   (b) Flooding
   (c) **Systematic desensitisation**
   (d) Addressing cognitive distortions
   (e) Homework exercises

This woman is experiencing agoraphobia with panic attacks. This can be a very debilitating condition and warrants urgent treatment. Systematic desensitisation is a behavioural component of cognitive–behavioural therapy that involves exposing the individual to perceived threat in a structured and graded way. Steps involved are establishing an 'anxiety stimulus hierarchy' (e.g. identifying which places make the patient anxious), learning a coping mechanism (e.g. pausing to use deep breathing exercises when feeling anxious) and finally, connecting the stimulus to the perceived threat (first visiting a small shop, then a larger one and finally the supermarket, using relaxation techniques at each step to connect a state of relaxation to the situation). See Beck (2011) and, for further reading, Rothbaum *et al* (2000).

9 A 19-year-old man says that he is 'scared to death' of spiders and cannot sleep at night, as he thinks there might be some in his room. When he last saw a spider, he became very frightened and felt he was going to faint. What psychological approach would be useful in treating this man?

    (a)   Psychoanalysis
    (b)   **Exposure and response prevention**
    (c)   Systematic desensitisation
    (d)   Addressing cognitive distortions
    (e)   Group therapy

This man has a specific phobia of spiders (also known as arachnophobia). Exposure and response prevention is a behavioural technique used for the treatment of phobias and OCD. A therapeutic effect is achieved as subjects confront their fears and discontinue their escape response. In this case, the patient could be exposed to a picture of a spider and advised not to look away or move away. He might then be able to cope with seeing a spider through habituation (a form of operant conditioning). In OCD, the equivalent of the escape response is the compulsive behaviour (e.g. excessive hand-washing), which is an abnormal coping mechanism for anxiety. See Beck (2011) and, for further reading, Huppert & Roth (2003).

10 A 21-year-old man becomes extremely distressed when his advances towards a woman in his university class are rejected. He feels it is very unfair that his feelings are not reciprocated as he cares deeply about her. He says that this always happens to him and that he has no hope of finding love in his life. He downplays the fact that two other women have expressed an interest in him. He believes that someone at his age should have a girlfriend. How would you categorise his thoughts in psychological terms?

    (a)   Immature thinking
    (b)   Extraversion
    (c)   Acting out
    (d)   **Cognitive distortions**
    (e)   Intellectualisation

The term cognitive distortion was coined by Aaron Beck to represent exaggerated or irrational thought patterns that lead to psychological problems, especially depression and anxiety. Targeting these distortions is a central component of cognitive–behavioural therapy.

This man is demonstrating a number of cognitive distortions, including fallacy of fairness, minimisation, all-or-nothing thinking and over-generalisation. See Grohol (2013) and, for further reading, Beck (1963) and Burns (1980).

11 A 37-year-old woman with a long-term history of depressive illness is referred to a psychologist for psychotherapy. The therapist encourages her to gain an understanding of the effect of her unconscious feelings on her relationships with her family. She also encourages her to make a connection between her past and present relationships. What type of therapy is being used here?

    (a)   Cognitive–behavioural therapy
    (b)   Interpersonal psychotherapy
    (c)   Cognitive analytical therapy
    (d)   **Psychodynamic psychotherapy**
    (e)   Schema therapy

Psychodynamic therapy (sometimes referred to as insight-oriented therapy) focuses on unconscious processes as they are manifested in a person's present behaviour. It is similar to psychoanalysis, in that it centres on the concepts that some maladaptive functioning in the present developed from earlier life experiences and that this maladaption is at least in part unconscious, and relies heavily on the interpersonal relationship between client and therapist. However, it is less intense than psychoanalysis, consisting of 50-min sessions once or twice a week.

The healing and change process envisioned in long-term psychodynamic therapy typically requires at least 2 years of sessions. Practitioners of brief psychodynamic therapy believe that some changes can happen through a more rapid process and tend to focus on one major psychological problem over a maximum of 25 sessions. See British Psychoanalytic Council (2004), Fonagy *et al* (2015) and Haggerty (2006).

12 A 21-year-old woman is preoccupied with her weight. She often binge-eats and subsequently causes herself to vomit. Her BMI is in the normal range. Which psychological treatments have been shown to be most effective for this condition?

    (a)   Psychoanalysis and cognitive–behavioural therapy (CBT)
    (b)   **CBT and interpersonal psychotherapy**
    (c)   Cognitive therapy and psychoanalysis
    (d)   Group therapy and supportive psychotherapy
    (e)   CBT and supportive psychotherapy

This woman has the eating disorder bulimia nervosa. NICE guidelines recommend the use of CBT specifically for bulimia nervosa (CBT-BN) and interpersonal psychotherapy as interventions. Both approaches were shown to be effective in a major Cochrane review. High-dose fluoxetine also has a role in treatment. See Hay *et al* (2009) and NICE (2004).

13 A 36-year-old man from Afghanistan describes intense 'reliving' of episodes of torture he experienced 10 years ago. He has nightmares about what happened to him and describes a heightened state of alert, especially at night while trying to sleep. He has begun to avoid public transport, as he was abducted while on a bus prior to his torture. What two types of psychological therapy are indicated for this man?

  (a) **Trauma-focused cognitive–behavioural therapy (CBT) and eye movement desensitisation and reprocessing (EMDR)**
  (b) Psychoanalysis and CBT
  (c) Debriefing and CBT
  (d) Interpersonal psychotherapy and EMDR
  (e) Supportive psychotherapy and psychoanalysis

This man has many of the core symptoms of PTSD – flashbacks, nightmares, hypervigilance, difficulty sleeping and avoidance behaviours. Trauma-focused CBT is a variant of CBT. It was initially developed for sexually abused children and their non-offending carers. It has been modified to assist those with all forms of PTSD and has been empirically demonstrated as an effective treatment. The therapist might ask the patient to confront their traumatic memories by thinking about their experience in detail. During this process, coping techniques are developed, while identifying any unhelpful thoughts or misrepresentations about the experience.

EMDR is a psychotherapy developed by Francine Shapiro that emphasises disturbing memories as the cause of PTSD psychopathology. According to Shapiro, when a traumatic or distressing experience occurs, the memory and associated stimuli are inadequately processed and stored in an isolated memory network. EMDR uses an eight-step protocol involving recollection of distressing images while receiving one of several types of bilateral sensory input, including side-to-side eye movements. It is thought that this process helps to unlock these distressing memories. It is supported by a considerable evidence base. See NHS Choices (2013) and, for further reading, Mannarino *et al* (2014) and Shapiro & Laliotis (2010).

EMI answers

Defence mechanisms

Options:

  (a) Splitting
  (b) Projection
  (c) Rationalisation
  (d) Regression
  (e) Repression
  (f) Reaction formation
  (g) Displacement
  (h) Dissociation

From the list above, choose the defence mechanism being used in each example.

1   A 25-year-old woman who is struggling in her job because of her drinking habits tells herself that the problem is her difficult boss. She denies that her drinking has increased in frequency and severity and also blames the commute to work for her problems.

(c) Rationalisation

2   A 65-year-old man is frustrated with his physical health difficulties and decreasing ability to engage in social activities. He becomes more and more irritable with his wife, who cannot understand this change in him.

(g) Displacement

3   A 15-year-old boy with separated parents who has been disruptive at school becomes angry with his mother, saying she is evil and he never wants to speak to her again. On the other hand, he tells her his father is a great Dad and would never treat him this way.

(a) Splitting

Choice of psychotherapy

Options:

- (a)   Cognitive–behavioural therapy
- (b)   Cognitive analytical therapy
- (c)   Dialectical behavioural therapy
- (d)   Interpersonal psychotherapy
- (e)   Psychodynamic psychotherapy
- (f)   Psychoanalysis
- (g)   Family therapy
- (h)   Grief counselling

From the list above, choose the most appropriate choice of therapy for each of the examples below. More than one therapy may be used for each scenario.

1   A 19-year-old woman with bulimia nervosa.

(a) Cognitive–behavioural therapy
(d) Interpersonal psychotherapy

2   A 22-year-old man demonstrating over-generalisation and somatisation.

(a) Cognitive–behavioural therapy

3   A 45-year-old woman with long-term relationship difficulties and a history of conflict in her family.

(e) Psychodynamic psychotherapy
(g) Family therapy

4   A 65-year-old man having a prolonged grief reaction and symptoms of depression following the death of his wife.

(d) Interpersonal psychotherapy
(h) Grief counselling

5   A 26-year-old man with emotionally unstable personality disorder and repeated self-harm.

(b) Cognitive analytical therapy
(c) Dialectical behavioural therapy

CHAPTER 11

Other topics

MCQs

Risk assessment

1 You are asked to assess a 19-year-old woman on a medical ward who has taken an overdose of paracetamol tablets. Which of the following is not an indicator of intent?

(a) Taking precautions against discovery
(b) Notifying a potential helper
(c) Drinking a volume of alcohol sufficient to impair judgement
(d) Leaving a suicide note
(e) Expression of dissatisfaction that attempt failed

2 You are asked to assess a 21-year-old man with a diagnosis of emotionally unstable (borderline) personality disorder in the emergency department. He has cut himself superficially on his arms. He says this was to 'relieve tension', that he did not intend to kill himself and that he feels better now. Which of the following is false?

(a) In this instance, suicidal intent was unlikely
(b) He should be offered support from services but does not necessarily require admission to hospital
(c) A full history is important
(d) In the long-term, he is less likely than those without a mental disorder to end his life
(e) Psychological therapy might be useful

3 You are asked by a family member of one of your patients about the risk of suicide in schizophrenia. Which of the following is true in relation to schizophrenia and suicide?

(a) The lifetime risk is about 1%
(b) Having a higher level of education is a protective factor
(c) Comorbid substance misuse is not related to risk of suicide
(d) Family history of suicide is not related to risk of suicide
(e) There is an increased risk with history of childhood trauma

4   You are asked to assess an 82-year-old man in the community who seems to be depressed. He is recently bereaved and lives by himself. His daughter is concerned that he wishes to end his life. Which of the following factors are not related to an increased risk of suicide in the elderly?

(a)   Older age
(b)   Female gender
(c)   Living alone
(d)   Bereavement
(e)   Depression

Forensic psychiatry

5   A 21-year-old man with a diagnosis of schizophrenia is arrested by police, having assaulted a member of the public in the street. On assessment, he seems intoxicated and psychotic. He has a history of assault. He is unemployed and has relationship difficulties. He was abused by his parents as a child. What is the greatest risk factor for future violence?

(a)   Psychotic illness
(b)   Substance misuse
(c)   History of violence
(d)   Relationship problems
(e)   Traumatic experiences

6   A 29-year-old man on an acute psychiatric ward is hostile and aggressive on the ward. Staff fear for their safety and that of the other patients and decide to use seclusion to contain the risk. Which of the following is true about use of seclusion in the UK?

(a)   Safety is the primary concern and ethical issues are not important
(b)   Seclusion is a very common practice in the UK
(c)   There is clear evidence that alternatives to seclusion are highly effective in acute management of violent patients
(d)   Alternatives to seclusion should always be considered in the first instance
(e)   Seclusion should be continued for 48 h before review

7   A 23-year-old man is arrested for exposing his erect penis to two women in a public place. Although he has not done this before, he admits he has had urges to do so over the past few years, which he finds distressing. How best is this behaviour classified?

(a)   Voyeurism
(b)   Sadomasochism
(c)   Frotteurism
(d)   Fetishism
(e)   Exhibitionism

8 A 17-year-old man with borderline intellectual disability repeatedly sets fires in his neighbourhood. He has set fire to trees, fences and advertising hoarding. He has been arrested for these but released without charge. There is no clear motive and he says that he does not know exactly why he does it, he 'just really likes fires'. He does not get aroused by setting the fires. He reads about fire departments and fire engines for hours each day online. What is the best clinical description of his behaviour?

(a) Arson
(b) Fire addiction
(c) Trichotillomania
(d) Vandalism
(e) Pathological fire-setting

Psychiatry in intellectual disability

9 A 5-year-old girl is accompanied to the clinic by her mother. The clinical notes state that she has a mild intellectual disability. Which of the following IQ ranges is consistent with a diagnosis of a mild intellectual disability?

(a) 90–99
(b) 70–89
(c) 50–69
(d) 35–49
(e) 20–34

10 A 20-year-old man with moderate intellectual disability is accompanied to the clinic by his mother. There has been a recent change in his behaviour. He has become more withdrawn and is eating less. His mother is worried that he might be depressed. All the following are true about the assessment for mental illness in people with intellectual disability, except?

(a) Mental disorders are overdiagnosed in intellectual disability
(b) Information from carers can aid diagnosis
(c) People with intellectual disability can have difficulty describing their symptoms
(d) The rate of mental disorder in intellectual disability is increased compared with the general population
(e) Assessment for physical problems should be performed

11 A 5-year-old boy is accompanied to the clinic by his father. He has Down syndrome and recently had an IQ assessment. His father wishes to discuss the diagnosis of Down syndrome with you. Which of the following is true regarding Down syndrome?

(a) It affects 1 in 10 newborn children
(b) In the majority of those affected, it is associated with severe to profound intellectual disability
(c) People with Down syndrome have increased rates of Alzheimer's disease
(d) Increased incidence with younger maternal age
(e) Normal life expectancy

12 A 22-year-old woman with a mild intellectual disability attends the out-patient clinic, accompanied by her carer. There has been a recent change in her behaviour: she has become more withdrawn and less socially active. All the following are principles of good clinical assessment in people with intellectual disability, except:

(a) History of the presenting complaint over time
(b) Assess for medical conditions
(c) Assess the person's level of understanding
(d) Exclude the carer from the assessment
(e) Assess for physical disabilities

Mental health law

13 A 45-year-old man with paranoid schizophrenia is detained under Section 3 of the Mental Health Act 1983 (as amended in 2007). Which of the following is not directly relevant to criteria for detention under the mental health act?

(a) The patient has paranoid schizophrenia
(b) The patient has threatened to assault his neighbour
(c) The patient has harmed himself in the past when he was unwell
(d) The patient refuses to take a depot injection
(e) The patient absolutely refuses to stay in hospital for treatment

14 A 23-year-old man with schizoaffective disorder detained under Section 3 of the Mental Health Act 1983 refuses to consent to treatment with antipsychotic medication. He is floridly psychotic, extremely agitated and aggressive and has threatened staff members and other patients on the ward. Which of the following is true?

(a) He cannot be treated as he has not given consent
(b) He can be treated because he is a psychiatric patient
(c) He can be treated as it is necessary to prevent serious deterioration, serious suffering or violence
(d) He can be treated because treatment is life-saving
(e) He should be discharged as he is not complying with the treatment plan

15 A 73-year-old woman with Alzheimer's disease is being assessed for capacity to consent to treatment. Which of the following is not required for her to have capacity?

(a) She must be able to understand the information given to her
(b) She must be able to retain this information long enough to make a decision
(c) She must be able to weigh up the information to inform her decision
(d) She must make a wise decision in keeping with the doctor's advice
(e) She must be able to communicate her decision

Transcultural psychiatry

16 Which of the following is not true about psychiatric illness across cultures?

(a) Psychiatric illness is not an invention of Western civilisation and is a major problem in other countries
(b) Rates of schizophrenia vary as much as 15–20% between different countries
(c) Cases of catatonia are more common in middle- and lower-income countries
(d) Conversion and dissociative disorders might be deemed normal behaviour in some cultures
(e) Anorexia nervosa is more common in higher-income countries

17 A 24-year-old man of Black ethnicity has recently been admitted to hospital with a first episode of psychosis. He presents with persecutory delusions, believing that the government wants to kill him and reports hearing voices informing him that he is in danger. He occasionally drinks alcohol and uses cannabis on 2–3 occasions per week. The following are all true in respect of psychosis in people from Black ethnic groups in the UK, except:

(a) Persecutory delusions are culturally appropriate
(b) Higher rates of psychosis compared with those of White ethnicity
(c) Smoking cannabis increases the risk of psychosis
(d) Higher rates of compulsory hospital admission
(e) Auditory hallucinations are a symptom of psychosis

18 Culture-bound syndromes are conditions with distinct symptom patterns that are unique to certain cultures. Which of the following is not a culture-bound syndrome?

(a) Koro
(b) Amok
(c) PTSD
(d) Arctic hysteria
(e) Locura

Professionalism and ethics

19 One of your colleagues has been accused of behaving in an 'unprofessional' manner at work and an internal investigation in the trust has been instigated. Which of the following is not a core component of medical professionalism?

(a) Professional competence
(b) Academic excellence
(c) Honesty with patients
(d) Patient confidentiality
(e) Improving quality of and access to care

20 You are very concerned about the behaviour of one of your fellow junior doctors on your psychiatry rotation. They are regularly intoxicated when coming to work. You mention this to your consultant, who is aware of the problem and has alerted the General Medical Council (GMC). Which of the following is not a core component of good medical practice according to GMC guidelines?

(a) Make the care of your patient your first concern
(b) Keep your professional knowledge and skills up to date
(c) Take prompt action if you think that patient safety, dignity or comfort is being compromised
(d) Work in partnership with patients
(e) Protect your colleagues first and foremost

21 One of the medical students attached to your firm seems stressed and tearful at a ward round. Your registrar takes time out to check if he is feeling all right. He suggests the student access the university mentorship programme and access counselling services to help cope with current stressors. Which of the following is not true about stress and burnout in medical students?

(a) Medical student well-being is affected by multiple stressors as well as positive aspects of medical training
(b) A student feeling pressure in medical school is unlikely to make a good doctor
(c) Attention to individual students' coping capacity can help promote well-being and minimise burnout
(d) Formal and informal offerings within medical schools can help develop coping capacity
(e) Helping students cultivate the skills to sustain their well-being throughout their careers has important payoffs for health services and patients

Patient-centred care

22 You are asked by a family member of one of your patients what is meant by the term 'recovery'. Which of the following would not be seen as an adequate summary of recovery by the recovery movement and service user groups?

(a) Overcoming the effects of being a patient in mental healthcare, and retaining or resuming some degree of control over one's own life

(b) Establishing a fulfilling, meaningful life and a positive sense of identity founded on hopefulness and self-determination

(c) A process of personal discovery of how to live (and how to live well) with enduring symptoms and vulnerabilities

(d) The absence of symptoms of mental illness and avoidance of admissions to hospital

(e) A way of living a satisfying, hopeful and contributing life even with limitations caused by the illness

23 At your weekly ward review, one of your patients attends with an advocate and brings a list of points of importance to their recovery. One of the items on the list reads 'to come off all medication'. Your consultant listens attentively to the patient and acknowledges that side-effects of medication can be difficult to deal with. She discusses the pros and cons of this with the patient and provides information to them in leaflet form about their illness and medications. She asks the patient to consider this information before they make a joint decision on the next step. What aspect of psychiatric practice is being demonstrated here?

(a) Working in partnership with patients

(b) Demonstration of empathy

(c) Psychoeducation

(d) Patient involvement

(e) All the above

EMI questions

Risk assessment

Options:

(a) History of violent behaviour

(b) Substance misuse problems

(c) No effort to conceal suicide attempt

(d) Depressive illness

(e) Psychotic illness

(f) Old age

(g) Female gender

(h) Dissocial personality disorder

Which of the above are:

1 Risk factors associated with violent behaviour (select 4 options)

2 Relative risk factors for suicide (select 4 options)

Mental health law

Options:

(a) Detention in hospital for up to 28 days
(b) The appointment of an individual to make decisions on the patient's behalf
(c) Detention in hospital for up to 12 months on first implementation
(d) The right to provide treatment for mental illness without consent where there is a risk to self or others
(e) Detention in hospital for treatment of physical health problems
(f) Results in decisions being made for the patient about all aspects of their life
(g) Detention in hospital for up to 6 months
(h) The right to provide treatment for mental illness without consent where there is no overt risk to the self or others
(i) Detention in hospital for assessment, but no right to treat without consent

Which of the above result from implementation of the following Acts, and which are not allowed?

1 Allowed by Section 2 of the Mental Health Act 1983 (select two options)

2 Allowed by Section 3 of the Mental Health Act 1983 (select two options)

3 Allowed by the Mental Capacity Act 2005 (select two options)

4 Not allowed by the Mental Health Act 1983 or Mental Capacity Act 2005 (select three options)

Professionalism and ethics

Options:

(a) A medical student presents a hospital case at a conference without obtaining patient consent
(b) A psychiatrist informs a colleague that a patient of his has threatened to harm them
(c) A woman reports thoughts of self-harm to a medical student, who then reports it to the psychiatrist
(d) A nurse is contacted by the local police by telephone and confirms, when asked, that a patient has a history of drug use
(e) A severely depressed patient informs the psychiatrist that he wishes to kill his wife; the psychiatrist then informs the patient's wife of this threat

(f) A patient with mania and loss of insight refuses antipsychotic medication, and is informed by their psychiatrist that they will receive intramuscular medication if they refuse oral medication

In the above scenarios, identify which of the following have occurred.

1 Inappropriate breaking of confidentiality (select two options)

2 Appropriate breaking of confidentiality (select three options)

MCQ answers

Risk assessment

1 You are asked to assess a 19-year-old woman on a medical ward who has taken an overdose of paracetamol tablets. Which of the following is not an indicator of intent?

    (a) Taking precautions against discovery
    (b) **Notifying a potential helper**
    (c) Drinking a volume of alcohol sufficient to impair judgement
    (d) Leaving a suicide note
    (e) Expressing dissatisfaction that attempt failed

The Becks' Suicide Intent Scale is a 21-item self-report questionnaire that can be used to identify the presence and severity of suicidal ideation. It was developed by Aaron T. Beck and his colleagues for use with patients who attempt suicide but survive. They recognised that it is important to understand a patient's will to die in order to assess the severity of the suicide attempt.

Notifying a potential helper is an indicator that the individual might not have wanted to die, and that the attempt might have represented a 'cry for help'. Although drinking a small volume of alcohol is a common occurrence in less serious attempts, a volume sufficient to diminish judgement is recognised as an indicator of increased intent, particularly if taken to facilitate the attempt. See Beck *et al* (1979).

2 You are asked to assess a 21-year-old man with a diagnosis of emotionally unstable (borderline) personality disorder in the emergency department. He has cut himself superficially on his arms. He says this was to 'relieve tension', that he did not intend to kill himself and that he feels better now. Which of the following is false?

    (a) In this instance, suicidal intent was unlikely
    (b) He should be offered support from services but does not necessarily require admission to hospital
    (c) A full history is important
    (d) **In the long-term, he is less likely than those without a mental disorder to end his life**
    (e) Psychological therapy might be useful

Suicidal behaviour is frequent in patients with emotionally unstable personality disorder (borderline personality disorder in DSM-5). At least 75% attempt suicide and approximately 10% eventually complete suicide

– a much higher proportion than in the general population. This is a very important point. It is a mistake to think a pattern of repeated self-harm or failed suicidal attempts indicates little desire to die. Borderline patients at greatest risk for suicidal behaviour include those with prior attempts, comorbid major depressive disorder, or a substance-use disorder.

On the other hand, deliberate self-harm such as superficial cutting is often carried out as a form of tension release and might serve as a form of emotion regulation. Dialectical behavioural therapy has been shown to be of benefit in managing deliberate self-harm in patients with emotionally unstable personality disorder. See Black *et al* (2004), Gratz (2003) and Stoffers *et al* (2012).

3   You are asked by a family member of one of your patients about the risk of suicide in schizophrenia. Which of the following is true in relation to schizophrenia and suicide?

    (a)   The lifetime risk is about 1%
    (b)   Having a higher level of education is a protective factor
    (c)   Comorbid substance misuse is not related to risk of suicide
    (d)   Family history of suicide is not related to risk of suicide
    (e)   **There is an increased risk with history of childhood trauma**

For decades, the estimated lifetime risk of suicide in patients with schizophrenia was 10%. However, recent studies and systematic reviews suggest that this rate is much lower – around 5%. Risk factors for later suicide include being young, being male and having a high level of education, a family history of suicide and comorbid substance misuse. The only consistent protective factor for suicide is delivery of and adherence to effective treatment. See Hor & Taylor (2010).

4   You are asked to assess an 82-year-old man in the community who seems to be depressed. He is recently bereaved and lives by himself. His daughter is concerned that he wishes to end his life. Which of the following factors are not related to an increased risk of suicide in the elderly?

    (a)   Older age
    (b)   **Female gender**
    (c)   Living alone
    (d)   Bereavement
    (e)   Depression

Despite the fact that suicide and its prevention continues to be a priority area for healthcare in the UK, suicide in the elderly remains under-researched. Suicide rates in most industrialised nations increase with age, the highest rates of all occurring in elderly men. Suicidal behaviour in the elderly is undertaken with greater intent and with greater lethality than in younger age groups. The notion that most elderly suicides are 'rational' acts in response to irreversible, understandable situations is not supported by available clinical research. Other risk factors in the elderly include psychiatric illness, alcohol misuse, previous suicide attempt, vulnerable personality traits, physical illness and pain. See Cattell (2000).

Forensic psychiatry

5 A 21-year-old man with a diagnosis of schizophrenia is arrested by police, having assaulted a member of the public in the street. On assessment, he seems intoxicated and psychotic. He has a history of assault. He is unemployed and has relationship difficulties. He was abused by his parents as a child. What is the greatest risk factor for future violence?

(a) Psychotic illness
(b) Substance misuse
(c) **History of violence**
(d) Relationship problems
(e) Traumatic experiences

The greatest predictor of future violence is past violence. According to his actuarial risk profile, this man would be deemed high risk, as he has several historical risk factors for violence. Risk management will need to focus on dynamic risk factors. See Eastman *et al* (2012) and, for further reading, Guy *et al* (2013).

6 A 29-year-old man on an acute psychiatric ward is hostile and aggressive on the ward. Staff fear for their safety and that of the other patients and decide to use seclusion to contain the risk. Which of the following is true about use of seclusion in the UK?

(a) Safety is the primary concern and ethical issues are not important
(b) Seclusion is a very common practice in the UK
(c) There is clear evidence that alternatives to seclusion are highly effective in acute management of violent patients
(d) **Alternatives to seclusion should always be considered in the first instance**
(e) Seclusion should be continued for 48 h before review

Seclusion (often referred to as supervised confinement) is a controversial topic in modern psychiatry. Despite widespread calls to end its use, it remains a reality in acute psychiatric wards, where it is used primarily to manage risk of serious violent incidents. Although many alternatives have been suggested, the evidence base to support their use in cases of acute aggression and violence is weak. Frequency varies significantly between countries, with the rate in the UK being quite low (0.05 incidents per day in acute psychiatric units, equivalent to one seclusion every 3 weeks). Seclusion is associated with aggression, alcohol use, absconding and medication refusal. Alternatives to seclusion, such as de-escalation, time out and as-needed medication should always be considered in the first instance. Seclusion is reviewed regularly, usually every 2 h by nursing staff and every 4 h by medical staff. See Bowers *et al* (2009) and Cleary *et al* (2010).

7   A 23-year-old man is arrested for exposing his erect penis to two women in a public place. Although he has not done this before, he admits he has had urges to do so over the past few years, which he finds distressing. How best is this behaviour classified?

(a)   Voyeurism
(b)   Sadomasochism
(c)   Frotteurism
(d)   Fetishism
(e)   **Exhibitionism**

Exhibitionism is classified as a disorder of sexual preference in ICD-10. In these disorders, there are recurrent, intense, sexual urges and fantasies involving unusual objects or activities. The person acts on the urges or is markedly distressed by them and the preference has been present for at least 6 months. Exhibitionism is defined as either a recurrent or a persistent tendency to expose one's genitalia to unsuspecting strangers (usually of the opposite sex), almost invariably associated with sexual arousal and masturbation. There is no intention or invitation to sexual intercourse with the 'witness(es)'. Exhibitionism has historically been viewed more as a nuisance than as a serious criminal justice matter. However, research has demonstrated that the number of exhibitionists who are detected reoffending is a significant under-representation of the number who actually reoffend. See WHO (1992).

8   A 17-year-old man with borderline intellectual disability repeatedly sets fires in his neighbourhood. He has set fire to trees, fences and advertising hoarding. He has been arrested for these but released without charge. There is no clear motive and he says that he does not know exactly why he does it, he 'just really likes fires'. He does not get aroused by setting the fires. He reads about fire departments and fire engines for hours each day online. What is the best clinical description of his behaviour?

(a)   Arson
(b)   Fire addiction
(c)   Trichotillomania
(d)   Vandalism
(e)   **Pathological fire-setting**

Pathological fire-setting (pyromania), as defined in ICD-10, is characterised by multiple acts of, or attempts at, setting fire to property or other objects, without apparent motive, and by a persistent preoccupation with subjects related to fire and burning. There might also be an abnormal interest in other things associated with fires, including calling out the fire service.

Arson is not a clinical diagnosis, but a crime defined as malicious, voluntary or wilful fire-setting to a building or property owned by another, or for an improper purpose, such as to collect insurance.

Pyromania is conceptualised differently in DSM-5. There, it is hallmarked by fascination with and attraction to fire and fire-starting paraphernalia, as well as the deliberate and repeated setting of fires. Individuals diagnosed with pyromania often experience tension or affective arousal before setting a fire, and feelings of pleasure, gratification, or relief during it or afterwards.

People who set fires are a heterogeneous group. Not all fire-setting behaviours result in a charge of arson and not all fire-setting is pathological. Psychiatric disorders can be present in fire-setters, however there is no direct relationship between any psychiatric disorder and arson. See Eastman *et al* (2012) and, for further reading, Doley (2003).

Psychiatry in intellectual disability

9   A 5-year-old girl is accompanied to the clinic by her mother. The clinical notes state that she has a mild intellectual disability. Which of the following IQ ranges is consistent with a diagnosis of a mild intellectual disability?

  (a)   90–99
  (b)   70–89
  (c)   **50–69**
  (d)   35–49
  (e)   20–34

'Learning disability' and 'intellectual disability' are the terms commonly used in clinical practice in the UK to describe people with a reduced level of intellectual functioning (IQ < 70) and a diminished ability to adapt to the daily demands of the normal social environment. The term 'mental retardation' is used in the ICD-10 classification manual, but is not used in clinical practice, as it is seen as a stigmatising, pejorative and inappropriate term. Intellectual disability is a descriptive concept, and not a disorder. Approximately 2% of the general population meet the criteria for an intellectual disability and approximately 96% have an IQ of 70–130.

The following IQ ranges are used to classify intellectual disability:

▶ mild disability: 50–69 (equivalent mental age 9–12 years)
▶ moderate disability: 35–49 (equivalent mental age 6–9 years)
▶ severe disability: 20–34 (equivalent mental age 3–6 years)
▶ profound disability: under 20 (equivalent mental age below 3 years).

See WHO (1992).

10 A 20-year-old man with moderate intellectual disability is accompanied to the clinic by his mother. There has been a recent change in his behaviour. He has become more withdrawn and is eating less. His mother is worried that he might be depressed. All the following are true about the assessment for mental illness in people with intellectual disability, except?

  (a)   **Mental disorders are overdiagnosed in intellectual disability**
  (b)   Information from carers can aid diagnosis
  (c)   People with intellectual disability can have difficulty describing their symptoms
  (d)   The rate of mental disorder in intellectual disability is increased compared with the general population
  (e)   Assessment for physical problems should be performed

The prevalence of mental disorders in intellectual disability is approximately 30–50%. Nonetheless, mental disorders are underdiagnosed. This might be due in part to diagnostic overshadowing – the tendency of clinicians to overlook comorbid mental disorder and to attribute changes in behaviour or ability to the intellectual disability. The description of symptoms can vary, depending on a person's language and communication skills and cognitive and intellectual ability, and is more difficult for those with moderate to severe intellectual disability. Detailed collateral information from a carer is an important component of the assessment.

Schizophrenia occurs in 3% of those with intellectual disability, compared with 1% of the general population. The incidence of bipolar affective disorder is increased 2- to 3-fold. Other common mental disorders in intellectual disability are depression, OCD, attention-deficit hyperactivity disorder, autism spectrum disorder and tic disorders. See Smiley (2005).

11 A 5-year-old boy is accompanied to the clinic by his father. He has Down syndrome and recently had an IQ assessment. His father wishes to discuss the diagnosis of Down syndrome with you. Which of the following is true regarding Down syndrome?

(a) It affects 1 in 10 newborn children
(b) In the majority of those affected, it is associated with severe to profound intellectual disability
(c) **People with Down syndrome have increased rates of Alzheimer's disease**
(d) Increased incidence with younger maternal age
(e) Normal life expectancy

The prognosis and life expectancy for people with Down syndrome has improved greatly in recent years, but still remains poorer than for the general population. However, this increasing life expectancy is associated with an increased rate of early-onset Alzheimer's disease. Approximately 75% of people with Down syndrome will develop symptoms of Alzheimer's disease during their lifetime.

Down syndrome is a common genetic cause of intellectual disability. It is primarily caused by trisomy of chromosome 21. It affects 1 in 500 of all conceptions and occurs in 1 in 1000 of live births. The incidence is increased with advancing maternal age. The IQ of people with Down syndrome is usually in the mild to moderate range on the intellectual disability spectrum (IQ range 35–69). See Stanton & Coetzee (2004).

12 A 22-year-old woman with a mild intellectual disability attends the out-patient clinic, accompanied by her carer. There has been a recent change in her behaviour: she has become more withdrawn and less socially active. All the following are principles of good clinical assessment in people with intellectual disability, except:

(a) History of the presenting complaint over time
(b) Assess for medical conditions
(c) Assess the person's level of understanding
(d) **Exclude the carer from the assessment**
(e) Assess for physical disabilities

Similar to all clinical assessments, a longitudinal history of the development of symptoms should be sought. The collateral information from a family member or a carer might be of extra importance in this case, particularly if the person has difficulty communicating. All efforts should be made to ascertain the patient's level of understanding and to frame information in a context they can understand. People with intellectual disability have increased rates of physical disability (e.g. hearing impairment) and comorbid medical conditions (e.g. epilepsy). They might have also have difficulty conveying to family or carers symptoms of any physical (e.g. pain) or mental (e.g. low mood) illness. See Allington-Smith (2006).

Mental health law

13 A 45-year-old man with paranoid schizophrenia is detained under Section 3 of the Mental Health Act 1983 (as amended in 2007). Which of the following is not directly relevant to criteria for detention under the mental health act?
   (a) The patient has paranoid schizophrenia
   (b) The patient has threatened to assault his neighbour
   (c) The patient has harmed himself in the past when he was unwell
   (d) **The patient refuses to take a depot injection**
   (e) The patient absolutely refuses to stay in hospital for treatment

The Mental Health Act 1983 has strict criteria for detention of patients in hospital. The most commonly used sections of the Act are Section 2, which allows detention for assessment for up to 28 days, and Section 3, which allows for detention for treatment for up to 6 months. The patient must have a mental disorder of sufficient nature or degree to require detention in hospital. Detention must be required for the patient's safety or the protection of others.

Section 3 also specifies that appropriate treatment must be available, and that the patient cannot be treated without section. Therefore if the patient refuses to stay in hospital and the treating team deem this is necessary, this suggests detention is required. Not wanting to take a depot or indeed any medication is not directly relevant to detention criteria, although it would be taken into account when assessing the overall clinical scenario.

Section 2 is often amended to Section 3 should the patient not be shown to improve in the assessment period. Section 3 may be renewed, first after 6 months and then annually, but this requires a hearing at an independent Mental Health Tribunal. A tribunal can also be requested at any time by the patient or their nearest relative.

14 A 23-year-old man with schizoaffective disorder detained under Section 3 of the Mental Health Act 1983 refuses to consent to treatment with antipsychotic medication. He is floridly psychotic, extremely agitated and aggressive and has threatened staff members and other patients on the ward. Which of the following is true?

(a) He cannot be treated as he has not given consent
(b) He can be treated because he is a psychiatric patient
(c) **He can be treated as it is necessary to prevent serious deterioration, serious suffering or violence**
(d) He can be treated because treatment is life-saving
(e) He should be discharged as he is not complying with the treatment plan

Patients' consent for treatment is required for all medical treatment except where that treatment is given under a specific legal power to treat without consent. There are clear guidelines in the Mental Health Act 1983 regarding consent to treatment. Consent-to-treat provisions refer to treatment for mental disorders only, and exclude psychosurgery and electroconvulsive therapy (for which there are different guidelines). In-patient treatment might be authorised by the approved clinician (usually the consultant psychiatrist). Exceptions to restrictions are when treatment is immediately necessary to save life, or non-irreversible, non-hazardous treatment is immediately necessary to prevent serious deterioration, serious suffering or violence.

15 A 73-year-old woman with Alzheimer's disease is being assessed for capacity to consent to treatment. Which of the following is not required for her to have capacity?

(a) She must be able to understand the information given to her
(b) She must be able to retain this information long enough to make a decision
(c) She must be able to weigh up the information to inform her decision
(d) **She must make a wise decision in keeping with the doctor's advice**
(e) She must be able to communicate her decision

The Mental Capacity Act 2005 was developed to give a clearer description of the concept of capacity referred to in clinical practice. Under the act, every person is assumed to have capacity until it is proven otherwise and there must be an identifiable reason for the alleged mental incapacity. If the person is deemed not to have capacity, a decision is made in their best interests. This is guided by the nearest relative or by someone nominated in an advance statement. Capacity is decision-specific – a person can have capacity to make one decision but not another – and can be fluctuating – a person can have capacity at one time but not at another. Decisions need not necessarily be wise or in agreement with conventional views. See Nicholson et al (2008).

Transcultural psychiatry

16 Which of the following is not true about psychiatric illness across cultures?

   (a) Psychiatric illness is not an invention of Western civilisation and is a major problem in other countries

   (b) **Rates of schizophrenia vary as much as 15–20% between different countries**

   (c) Cases of catatonia are more common in middle- and lower-income countries

   (d) Conversion and dissociative disorders might be deemed normal behaviour in some cultures

   (e) Anorexia nervosa is more common in higher-income countries

Psychiatric illnesses exist throughout the world. Although there is fluctuation in the rates of certain conditions, the incidence of major mental illness such as schizophrenia does not vary widely between countries. Cultural factors are very important in interpreting signs and symptoms of mental illness and differences in non-verbal communication and belief systems might be misinterpreted if not closely considered. Conversion and dissociative disorders are more common in some cultures, where physical manifestations of mental distress are more common and might be deemed culturally normal. Anorexia nervosa is more common in higher-income countries, where strong cultural influences promote thinness as the ideal body shape. See Semple & Smyth (2013b).

17 A 24-year-old man of Black ethnicity has recently been admitted to hospital with a first episode of psychosis. He presents with persecutory delusions, believing that the government wants to kill him and reports hearing voices informing him that he is in danger. He occasionally drinks alcohol and uses cannabis on 2–3 occasions per week. The following are all true in respect of psychosis in people from Black ethnic groups in the UK, except:

   (a) **Persecutory delusions are culturally appropriate**

   (b) Higher rates of psychosis compared with those of White ethnicity

   (c) Smoking cannabis increases the risk of psychosis

   (d) Higher rates of compulsory hospital admission

   (e) Auditory hallucinations are a symptom of psychosis

The incidence of psychotic disorders is increased in many immigrant groups around the world. In the UK, the most elevated risk has been found for those of African-Caribbean and Black African ethnicity. Ethnic disparities in mental healthcare provision and outcomes continue to be of concern in the UK, with people of Black ethnicity having more adverse pathways to care, including an increased rate of hospital detention under the Mental Health Act 1983, police involvement with hospital admission, and more frequent hospital readmissions. These replicated findings continue to be a source of controversy and have led some to question the existence of institutional racism in mental health services.

    The rates of psychosis are higher for second- and third-generation immigrants from these ethnic groups than in first-generation immigrants.

Possible explanations for the higher rates of psychosis in Black ethnic groups compared with White ethnic groups include a higher burden of social adversity, a consequence of increased urbanicity, and increased cultural assimilation problems for later-generation immigrants.

Delusions are a symptom of psychosis and not culturally approved beliefs that someone might have. There is no evidence that paranoid beliefs are culturally sanctioned in some ethnic groups more so than others. Smoking cannabis has been associated with increased rates of psychosis, regardless of ethnic background. See Morgan *et al* (2010) and Sharpley *et al* (2001).

18 Culture-bound syndromes are conditions with distinct symptom patterns that are unique to certain cultures. Which of the following is not a culture-bound syndrome?

   (a)   Koro
   (b)   Amok
   (c)   **PTSD**
   (d)   Arctic hysteria
   (e)   Locura

PTSD is an internationally recognised condition related to severe traumatic experience. It might be more common in certain countries, where war and natural disaster have affected large proportions of the population. The other conditions listed are recognised culture-bound syndromes. Koro (Malaysia) refers to the belief that the genitals are retreating into the abdomen. Amok (Malay men) refers to sudden, unprovoked acts of violence followed by suicide. Pibloko (Polar Eskimo women) or 'Arctic hysteria' is a dissociative state resulting from personal loss. Locura (Latin America) is a severe form of chronic psychosis attributed to adverse life events and personal vulnerability. See Semple & Smyth (2013*b*).

Professionalism and ethics

19 One of your colleagues has been accused of behaving in an 'unprofessional' manner at work and an internal investigation in the trust has been instigated. Which of the following is not a core component of medical professionalism?

   (a)   Professional competence
   (b)   **Academic excellence**
   (c)   Honesty with patients
   (d)   Patient confidentiality
   (e)   Improving quality of and access to care

Professionalism has become a matter of increasing importance in modern times. Guidelines for professionalism have been outlined by several governing bodies and are important to be aware of for all doctors. Although keeping up to date with clinical and scientific knowledge is vitally important for patient care, academic achievement is not necessarily a measure of good professional practice. See Bhugra & Gupta (2010).

20 You are very concerned about the behaviour of one of your fellow junior doctors on your psychiatry rotation. They are regularly intoxicated when coming to work. You mention this to your consultant, who is aware of the problem and has alerted the General Medical Council (GMC). Which of the following is not a core component of good medical practice according to GMC guidelines?

(a) Make the care of your patient your first concern
(b) Keep your professional knowledge and skills up to date
(c) Take prompt action if you think that patient safety, dignity or comfort is being compromised
(d) Work in partnership with patients
(e) **Protect your colleagues first and foremost**

Being intoxicated on duty is highly unprofessional and jeopardises patient care. In this instance, you are correct to raise this matter with your senior colleague. Your more experienced colleague will be better placed to escalate the matter to the level of investigation required – in this case, the GMC. See GMC (2013).

21 One of the medical students attached to your firm seems stressed and tearful at a ward round. Your registrar takes time out to check if he is feeling all right. He suggests the student access the university mentorship programme and access counselling services to help cope with current stressors. Which of the following is not true about stress and burnout in medical students?

(a) Medical student well-being is affected by multiple stressors as well as positive aspects of medical training
(b) **A student feeling pressure in medical school is unlikely to make a good doctor**
(c) Attention to individual students' coping capacity can help promote well-being and minimise burnout
(d) Formal and informal offerings within medical schools can help develop coping capacity
(e) Helping students cultivate the skills to sustain their well-being throughout their careers has important payoffs for health services and patients

Stress and burnout are important issues for medical students and doctors. Ignoring problems can lead to negative and even tragic consequences for students, doctors and patients. There is no evidence to suggest that a student feeling stress will not make a good doctor, although if not addressed, it could lead to burnout. Early intervention and peer and mentorship support is very important. See Dunn *et al* (2008).

Patient-centred care

22 You are asked by a family member of one of your patients what is meant by the term 'recovery'. Which of the following would not be seen as an adequate summary of recovery by the recovery movement and service user groups?

   (a)   Overcoming the effects of being a patient in mental healthcare, and retaining or resuming some degree of control over one's own life
   (b)   Establishing a fulfilling, meaningful life and a positive sense of identity founded on hopefulness and self-determination
   (c)   A process of personal discovery of how to live (and how to live well) with enduring symptoms and vulnerabilities
   (d)   **The absence of symptoms of mental illness and avoidance of admissions to hospital**
   (e)   A way of living a satisfying, hopeful and contributing life even with limitations caused by the illness

In recent years, the concept of recovery from severe mental illness has increasingly gained relevance in psychiatry. Countries all over the world have introduced recovery policy into mental health services. However, there is still debate about the concept, such as whether symptom reduction is central or not. In the 'service-based' definition of recovery, remission is defined as an improvement in symptoms and other deficits to a degree that they would be considered within a normal range, whereas recovery can be seen as a long-term goal of remission.

A second definition of recovery came from the self-help and consumer/user/survivor movement. Here, recovery can include, but does not require, symptom remission or a return to normal functioning. Recovery is seen as a process of personal growth and development, and involves overcoming the effects of being a mental health patient, with all its implications, to regain control and establish a personally fulfilling, meaningful life. It is critically important for modern psychiatrists to be aware of these alternative viewpoints, which sometimes cause friction, although they need not be mutually exclusive. See Schrank & Slade (2007).

23 At your weekly ward review, one of your patients attends with an advocate and brings a list of points of importance to their recovery. One of the items on the list reads 'to come off all medication'. Your consultant listens attentively to the patient and acknowledges that side-effects of medication can be difficult to deal with. She discusses the pros and cons of this with the patient and provides information to them in leaflet form about their illness and medications. She asks the patient to consider this information before they make a joint decision on the next step. What aspect of psychiatric practice is being demonstrated here?

   (a)   Working in partnership with patients
   (b)   Demonstration of empathy
   (c)   Psychoeducation
   (d)   Patient involvement
   (e)   **All the above**

Patient involvement in the planning and provision of mental health services has been growing over the past two decades in many countries. The ethical argument for patient involvement is based on principles such as autonomy, continuity, accessibility, accountability, and efficiency. There is also evidence that patient involvement in research and service development can make essential contributions, for example in identifying unmet needs, improving quality of life and guiding practice on contentious issues such as electroconvulsive therapy.

Psychoeducation is considered very important in modern psychiatry and has been shown to be effective in management of bipolar affective disorder. However, a review by Lincoln *et al* (2007) highlighted its limitations and stressed the importance of family involvement and the development of an evidence base. See Lincoln *et al* (2007), Smith *et al* (2010) and Thornicroft & Tansella (2005).

EMI answers

Risk assessment

Options:

- (a) History of violent behaviour
- (b) Substance misuse problems
- (c) No effort to conceal suicide attempt
- (d) Depressive illness
- (e) Psychotic illness
- (f) Old age
- (g) Female gender
- (h) Dissocial personality disorder

Which of the above are:

1 Risk factors associated with violent behaviour (select 4 options)

(a) History of violent behaviour
(b) Substance misuse problems
(e) Psychotic illness
(h) Dissocial personality disorder

2 Relative risk factors for suicide (select 4 options)

(b) Substance misuse problems
(d) Depressive illness
(e) Psychotic illness
(f) Old age

Mental health law

Options:

- (a) Detention in hospital for up to 28 days
- (b) The appointment of an individual to make decisions on the patient's behalf
- (c) Detention in hospital for up to 12 months on first implementation
- (d) The right to provide treatment for mental illness without consent where there is a risk to self or others
- (e) Detention in hospital for treatment of physical health problems
- (f) Results in decisions being made for the patient about all aspects of their life
- (g) Detention in hospital for up to 6 months
- (h) The right to provide treatment for mental illness without consent where there is no overt risk to the self or others
- (i) Detention in hospital for assessment, but no right to treat without consent

Which of the above result from implementation of the following Acts, and which are not allowed?

1 Allowed by Section 2 of the Mental Health Act 1983 (select 2 options)

(a) Detention in hospital for up to 28 days

(i) Detention in hospital for assessment, but not right to treat without consent

2 Allowed by Section 3 of the Mental Health Act 1983 (select 2 options)

(d) The right to provide treatment for mental illness without consent where there is a risk to self or others

(g) Detention in hospital for up to 6 months

3 Allowed by the Mental Capacity Act 2005 (select 2 options)

(b) The appointment of an individual to make decisions on the patient's behalf

(e) Detention in hospital for treatment of physical health problems

4 Not allowed by the Mental Health Act 1983 or Mental Capacity Act 2005 (select 3 options)

(c) Detention in hospital for up to 12 months on first implementation

(f) Results in decisions being made for the patient about all aspects of their life

(h) The right to provide treatment for mental illness without consent where there is no overt risk to the self or others

Professionalism and ethics

Options:

(a) A medical student presents a hospital case at a conference without obtaining patient consent

(b) A psychiatrist informs a colleague that a patient of his has threatened to harm them

(c) A woman reports thoughts of self-harm to a medical student, who then reports it to the psychiatrist

(d) A nurse is contacted by the local police by telephone and confirms, when asked, that a patient has a history of drug use

(e) A severely depressed patient informs the psychiatrist that he wishes to kill his wife; the psychiatrist then informs the patient's wife of this threat

(f) A patient with mania and loss of insight refuses antipsychotic medication, and is informed by their psychiatrist that they will receive intramuscular medication if they refuse oral medication

In the above scenarios, identify which of the following have occurred.

1 Inappropriate breaking of confidentiality (select two options)

(a) A medical student presents a hospital case at a conference without obtaining patient consent

(d) A nurse is contacted by the local police by telephone and confirms, when asked, that a patient has a history of drug use

2 Appropriate breaking of confidentiality (select three options)

(b) A psychiatrist informs a colleague that a patient of his has threatened to harm them

(c) A woman reports thoughts of self-harm to a medical student, who then reports it to the psychiatrist

(e) A severely depressed patient informs the psychiatrist that he wishes to kill his wife; the psychiatrist then informs the patient's wife of this threat

References

Afari N, Buchwald D (2003) Chronic fatigue syndrome: a review. *American Journal of Psychiatry*, **160**: 221–36.

Agrawal N, Govender S (2011) Epilepsy and neuropsychiatric comorbidities. *Advances in Psychiatric Treatment*, **17**: 44–53.

Ahmed AS (2007) Post-traumatic stress disorder, resilience and vulnerability. *Advances in Psychiatric Treatment*, **13**: 369–75.

Ahuja N, Cole AJ (2009) Hyperthermia syndromes in psychiatry. *Advances in Psychiatric Treatment*, **15**: 181–91.

Alberti KG, Zimmet P, Shaw J (2006) Metabolic syndrome – a new world-wide definition. A Consensus Statement from the International Diabetes Federation. *Diabetic Medicine*, **23**: 469–80.

Allington-Smith P (2006) Mental health of children with learning disabilities. *Advances in Psychiatric Treatment*, **12**: 130–8.

Alzheimer's Association (n.d.) *New Diagnostic Criteria and Guidelines for Alzheimer's Disease* (http://www.alz.org/research/diagnostic_criteria).

Alzheimer's Association (2013) 2013 Alzheimer's disease facts and figures. *Alzheimer's and Dementia*, **9**: 208–45.

American Psychiatric Association (2013) *Diagnostic and Statistical Manual of Mental Disorders (5th edn)*. APA.

Antshel KM, Hargrave TM, Simonescu M, *et al* (2011) Advances in understanding and treating ADHD. *BMC Medicine*, **9**: 72.

Arseneault L, Cannon M, Witton J, *et al* (2004) Causal association between cannabis and psychosis: examination of the evidence. *British Journal of Psychiatry*, **184**: 110–7.

Baddeley A (2003) Working memory and language: an overview. *Journal of Communication Disorders*, **36**: 189–208.

Baldwin R (2008) Depressive disorders. In *Oxford Textbook of Old Age Psychiatry* (eds R Jacoby, C Oppenheimer, T Denning, *et al*). Oxford University Press.

Bak M, Fransen A, Janssen J, *et al* (2014) Almost all antipsychotics result in weight gain: a meta-analysis. *PLoS ONE*, **9**: e94112.

Barbui C, Signoretti A, Mule S, *et al* (2009) Does the addition of a second antipsychotic drug improve clozapine treatment? *Schizophrenia Bulletin*, **35**: 458–68.

Barr Taylor C (2006) Panic disorder. *BMJ*, **332**: 951–5.

Bauer M, Pfenning A, Severus E, *et al* (2013) World Federation of Societies of Biological Psychiatry (WFSBP) guidelines for biological treatment of unipolar depressive disorders, part 1: update 2013 on the acute and continuation treatment of unipolar depressive disorders. *World Journal of Biolological Psychiatry*, **14**: 334–85.

Beck AT (1963) Thinking and depression: I. Idiosyncratic content and cognitive distortions. *Archives of General Psychiatry*, **9**: 324–33.

Beck JS (2011) *Cognitive Behavior Therapy: Basics and Beyond*. Guilford Press.

Beck AT, Kovacs M, Weissman A (1979) Assessment of suicidal intention: the Scale for Suicide Ideation. *Journal of Consulting and Clinical Psychology*, **47**: 343–52.

Bhugra D, Gupta S (2010) Medical professionalism in psychiatry. *Advances in Psychiatric Treatment*, **16**: 10–13.

Bhugra D, McKenzie K (2003) Expressed emotion across cultures. *Advances in Psychiatric Treatment*, **9**: 342–8.

Black DW, Blum N, Pfohl B, *et al* (2004) Suicidal behavior in borderline personality disorder: prevalence, risk factors, prediction, and prevention. *Journal of Personality Disorders*, **18**: 226–39.

Bowers L, van der Merwe M, Nijman H, *et al* (2009) The practice of seclusion and timeout on English acute psychiatric wards: the City-128 Study. *Archives of Psychiatric Nursing*, **24**: 275–86.

Bowlby J (1999) *Attachment: Attachment and Loss*, vol. 1 (2nd edn). Basic Books.

Brandt F, Thvilum M, Almind D, *et al* (2014) Hyperthyroidism and psychiatric morbidity: evidence from a Danish nationwide register study. *European Journal of Endocrinology*, **170**: 341–8.

Brewer, JA, Potenza MN (2008) The neurobiology and genetics of impulse control disorders: relationships to drug addictions. *Biochemical Pharmacology*, **75**: 63–75.

British Psychoanalytic Council (2004) *Making Sense of Psychotherapy and Psychoanalysis*. British Psychoanalytic Council and Mind.

Brown SA, Inaba RK, Gillin JC, *et al* (1995) Alcoholism and affective disorder: clinical course of depressive symptoms. *American Journal of Psychiatry*, **152**: 45–52.

Buchanan RW (2007) Persistent negative symptoms in schizophrenia: an overview. *Schizophrenia Bulletin*, **33**: 1013–22.

Buckley PF, Wirshing DA, Bhushan P, *et al* (2007) Lack of insight in schizophrenia. *CNS Drugs*, **21**: 129–41.

Bulik CM, Berkman ND, Brownley KA, *et al* (2007) Anorexia nervosa treatment: a systematic review of randomized controlled trials. *International Journal of Eating Disorders*, **40**: 310–20.

Burcusa SL, Iacono WG (2007) Risk for recurrence in depression. *Clinical Psychology Review*, **27**: 959–85.

Burns DD (1980) *Feeling Good: The New Mood Therapy*. New American Library.

Bushe C, Yeomans D, Floyd T, *et al* (2008) Categorical prevalence and severity of hyperprolactinaemia in two UK cohorts of patients with severe mental illness during treatment with antipsychotics. *Journal of Psychopharmacology*, **22**: 56–62.

Cattell H (2000) Suicide in the elderly. *Advances in Psychiatric Treatment*, **6**: 102–8.

Cermolacce M, Sass L, Parnas J (2010) What is bizarre in bizarre delusions? A critical review. *Schizophrenia Bulletin*, **36**: 667–9.

Chang C-K, Hayes RD, Perera G, *et al* (2011) Life expectancy at birth for people with serious mental illness and other major disorders from a secondary mental healthcare case register in London. *PLoS One*, **6**: e19590.

Chemerinski E, Triebwasser J, Roussos P, *et al* (2013) Schizotypal personality disorder. *Journal of Personality Disorders*, **27**: 652–79.

Choi H, Morrell MJ (2003) Review of lamotrigine and its clinical applications in epilepsy. *Expert Opinion on Pharmacotherapy*, **4**: 243–51.

Christensen J, Vestergaard M, Mortensen PB, *et al* (2007) Epilepsy and risk of suicide: a population-based case–control study. *Lancet Neurology*, **6**: 693–8.

Cleary M, Hunt GE, Walter G (2010) Seclusion and its context in acute inpatient psychiatric care. *Journal of Medical Ethics*, **36**: 459–62.

Cormac I, Brown A, Creasey S, *et al* (2010) A retrospective evaluation of the impact of total smoking cessation on psychiatric inpatients taking clozapine. *Acta Psychiatrica Scandinavica*, **121**: 393–7.

Cowen P, Harrison P, Burns T (2012) *Shorter Oxford Textbook of Psychiatry* (6th edn). Oxford University Press.

Cramer P (2000) Defense mechanisms in psychology today: Further processes for adaptation. *American Psychologist*, **55**: 637.

David A, Fleminger S, Kopelman M, *et al* (eds) (2009) *Lishman's Organic Psychiatry: A Textbook of Neuropsychiatry* (4th edn). Wiley–Blackwell.

De Hert M, Cohen D, Bobes J, *et al* (2011*a*) Physical illness in patients with severe mental disorders. II. Barriers to care, monitoring and treatment guidelines, plus recommendations at the system and individual level. *World Psychiatry*, **10**: 138–51.

De Hert M, Correll CU, Bobes J, *et al* (2011*b*) Physical illness in patients with severe mental disorders. I. Prevalence, impact of medications and disparities in health care. *World Psychiatry*, **10**: 52–77.

Derenne JL, Baldessarini RJ (2005) Clozapine toxicity associated with smoking cessation: case report. *American Journal of Therapeutics*, **12**: 469–71.

Doley R (2003) Pyromania: fact or fiction? *British Journal of Criminology*, **43**: 797–807.

Drake RE, Ehrlich J (1985) Suicide attempts associated with akathisia. *American Journal of Psychiatry*, **142**: 499–501.

Dunn LB, Iglewicz A, Moutier C (2008) A conceptual model of medical student well-being: promoting resilience and preventing burnout. *Academic Psychiatry*, **32**: 44–53.

Dutta R, Murray RM, Hotopf M, *et al* (2010) Reassessing the long-term risk of suicide after a first episode of psychosis. *Archives of General Psychiatry*, **67**: 1230–7.

Eastman N, Adshead G, Fox S, *et al* (2012) *Forensic Psychiatry*. Oxford University Press.

Feldman HM, Reiff MI (2014) Attention deficit–hyperactivity disorder in children and adolescents. *New England Journal of Medicine*, **370**: 838–46.

Ferguson JM (2001) SSRI antidepressant medications: adverse effects and tolerability. *Primary Care Companion – Journal of Clinical Psychiatry*, **3**: 22–7.

Fineberg N, Brown A (2011) Pharmacotherapy for obsessive–compulsive disorder. *Advances in Psychiatric Treatment*, **17**: 419–34.

Fleminger S (2009) Head injury. In *Lishman's Organic Psychiatry: A Textbook of Neuropsychiatry* (4th edn) (eds A David, S Fleminger, M Kopelman, *et al*). Wiley–Blackwell.

Folstein MF, Folstein SE, McHugh PR (1975) Mini-Mental State. A practical method for grading the cognitive state of patients for the clinician. *Journal of Psychiatric Research*, **12**: 189–98.

Fonagy P, Rost F, Carlyle JA (2015) Pragmatic randomized controlled trial of long-term psychoanalytic psychotherapy for treatment-resistant depression: the Tavistock Adult Depression Study (TADS). *World Psychiatry*, **14**: 312–21.

Frank E, Thase ME (1999) Natural history and preventative treatment of recurrent mood disorders. *Annual Review of Medicine*, **50**: 453–68.

Fukuda K, Straus SE, Hickie I, *et al* (1994) The chronic fatigue syndrome: a comprehensive approach to its definition and study. International Chronic Fatigue Syndrome Study Group. *Annals of Internal Medicine*, **121**: 953–9.

Fuller RK, Gordis E (2004) Does disulfiram have a role in alcoholism treatment today? *Addiction*, **99**: 21–4.

General Medical Council (2013) *Good Medical Practice*. GMC.

Gervin M, Barnes TRE (2000) Assessment of drug-related movement disorders in schizophrenia. *Advances in Psychiatric Treatment*, **6**: 332–41.

Gleason A, Castle D (2012) Adult attention-deficit hyperactivity disorder and bipolar disorder. *Advances in Psychiatric Treatment*, **18**: 198–204.

Glenn AL, Raine A (2011) Antisocial personality disorders. In *The Oxford Handbook of Social Neuroscience* (eds J Decety, JT Cacioppo). Oxford University Press.

Godlee F, Smith J, Marcovitch H (2011) Wakefield's article linking MMR vaccine and autism was fraudulent. *BMJ*, **342**: c7452.

Gogtay N, Rapoport J (2008) Clozapine use in children and adolescents. *Expert Opinion on Pharmacotherapy*, **9**: 459–65.

Goldstein BJ, Goodnick PJ (1998) Selective serotonin reuptake inhibitors in the treatment of affective disorders – III. Tolerability, safety and pharmacoeconomics. *Journal of Psychopharmacology*, **12**: S55–87.

Gratz KL (2003) Risk factors for and functions of deliberate self-harm: An empirical and conceptual review. *Clinical Psychology: Science and Practice*, **10**: 192–205.

Green B (2013) Post-traumatic stress disorder: new directions in pharmacotherapy. *Advances in Psychiatric Treatment*, **19**: 181–90.

Greenberg DM, Lee JW (2001) Psychotic manifestations of alcoholism. *Current Psychiatry Reports*, **3**: 314–8.

Grohol JM (2013) 15 common cognitive distortions. *Psych Central* (http://psychcentral.com/lib/15-common-cognitive-distortions/0002153).

Gunes A, Bilir E, Zenfil H, *et al* (2007) Inhibitory effect of valproic acid on cytochrome P450 2C9 activity in epilepsy patients. *Basic and Clinical Pharmacology and Toxicology*, **100**: 383–6.

Gurrera RJ, Caroff SN, Cohen A, *et al* (2011) An international consensus study of neuroleptic malignant syndrome diagnostic criteria using the Delphi method. *Journal of Clinical Psychiatry*, **72**: 1222–8.

Guy LS, Wilson CM, Douglas KS, *et al* (2013) *HCR-20 Version 3: Item-By-Item Summary of Violence Literature. HCR-20 Violence Risk Assessment White Paper Series, 3*. Simon Fraser University.

Haddad PM, Wieck A (2004) Antipsychotic-induced hyperprolactinaemia: mechanisms, clinical features and management. *Drugs*, **64**: 2291–314.

Haggerty J (2006) Psychodynamic therapy. *Psych Central* (http://psychcentral.com/lib/psychodynamic-therapy/000119).

Hansen L (2001) A critical review of akathisia, and its possible association with suicidal behaviour. *Human Psychopharmacology*, **16**: 495–505.

Hare RD, Vertommen H (2003) *The Hare Psychopathy Checklist – Revised*. Multi-Health Systems.

Harper RG (2010) Paranoid personality disorder. In *Corsini Encyclopedia of Psychology* (eds IB Weiner, WE Craighead). Wiley.

Harrison NA, Kopelman MD (2009) Endocrine diseases and metabolic disorders. In *Lishman's Organic Psychiatry: A Textbook of Neuropsychiatry* (eds AS David, S Fleminger, MD Kopelman, *et al*). Wiley–Blackwell.

Hay PP, Bacaltchuk J, Stefano S, *et al* (2009) Psychological treatments for bulimia nervosa and binging. *Cochrane Database of Systematic Reviews*, **7**: CD000562.

Hill P (2015) Attention-deficit hyperactivity disorder in children and adolescents: assessment and treatment. *Advances in Psychiatric Treatment*, **21**: 23–30.

Hinney A, Volckmar AL (2013) Genetics of eating disorders. *Current Psychiatry Reports*, **15**: 1–9.

Hoge EA, Ivkovic A, Fricchione GL (2012) Generalized anxiety disorder: diagnosis and treatment. *BMJ*, **345**: e7500.

Hogg J (2008) *Delirium*. In *Oxford Textbook of Old Age Psychiatry* (eds R Jacoby, C Oppenheimer, T Denning, *et al*). Oxford University Press.

Hor K, Taylor M (2010) Suicide and schizophrenia: a systematic review of rates and risk factors. *Journal of Psychopharmacology*, **24** (Suppl): 81–90.

Hornberger M, Piguet O (2012) Episodic memory in frontotemporal dementia: a critical review. *Brain*, **135**: 678–92.

Howard R (2008) Late onset schizophrenia and very late onset schizophrenia-like psychosis. In *Oxford Textbook of Old Age Psychiatry* (eds R Jacoby, C Oppenheimer, T Denning, *et al*). Oxford University Press.

Howes OD, Murray RM (2014) Schizophrenia: an integrated sociodevelopmental-cognitive model. *Lancet*, **383**: 1677–87.

Huppert JD, Roth D (2003) Treating obsessive–compulsive disorder with exposure and response prevention. *The Behavior Analyst Today*, **4**: 66–70.

Iancu I, Lowengrub K, Dembinsky Y, *et al* (2008) Pathological gambling: an update on neuropathophysiology and pharmacotherapy. *CNS Drugs*, **22**: 123–38.

Jaaskelainen E, Juola P, Hirvonen N, *et al* (2013) A systematic review and meta-analysis of recovery in schizophrenia. *Schizophrenia Bulletin*, **39**: 1296–306.

Jacob S, Spinler SA (2006) Hyponatremia associated with selective serotonin-reuptake inhibitors in older adults. *Annals of Pharmacotherapy*, **40**: 1618–622.

James L, Barnes TR, Lelliott P, *et al* (2007) Informing patients of the teratogenic potential of mood stabilizing drugs: a case note review of the practice of psychiatrists. *Journal of Psychopharmacology*, **21**: 815–9.

Jauhar S, McKenna PJ, Radua J, *et al* (2014) Cognitive–behavioural therapy for the symptoms of schizophrenia: systematic review and meta-analysis with examination of potential bias. *British Journal of Psychiatry*, **204**: 20–29.

Jelicic M, Ceunen E, Peters MJ, *et al* (2011) Detecting coached feigning using the Test of Memory Malingering (TOMM) and the Structured Inventory of Malingered Symptomatology (SIMS). *Journal of Clinical Psychology*, **67**: 850–55.

Joint Formulary Committee (2014) *British National Formulary (67)*. BMJ Group & Pharmaceutical Press.

Jones I, Smith S (2009) Puerperal psychosis: identifying and caring for women at risk. *Advances in Psychiatric Treatment*, **15**: 411–18.

Jones PB, Barnes TR, Davies L, *et al* (2006) Randomized controlled trial of the effect on Quality of Life of second- vs first-generation antipsychotic drugs in schizophrenia: Cost Utility of the Latest Antipsychotic Drugs in Schizophrenia Study (CUtLASS 1). *Archives of General Psychiatry*, **63**: 1079–87.

Jones WR, Morgan JF, Arcelus J (2013) Managing physical risk in anorexia nervosa. *Advances in Psychiatric Treatment*, **19**: 201–2.

Jung CG (1961) *Memories, Dreams, Reflections*. Vintage.

Kane JM, Correll CU, Goff DC, *et al* (2009) A multicenter, randomized, double-blind, placebo-controlled, 16-week study of adjunctive aripiprazole for schizophrenia or schizoaffective disorder inadequately treated with quetiapine or risperidone monotherapy. *Journal of Clinical Psychiatry*, **70**: 1348–57.

Kapur S, Zipursky R, Jones C, *et al* (2000) Relationship between dopamine D(2) occupancy, clinical response, and side effects: a double-blind PET study of first-episode schizophrenia. *American Journal of Psychiatry*, **157**: 514–20.

Keel PK, Forney KJ (2013) Psychosocial risk factors for eating disorders. *International Journal of Eating Disorders*, **46**: 433–9.

Kendall T, Pilling S, Tyrer P, *et al* (2009) Borderline and antisocial personality disorders: summary of NICE guidance. *BMJ*, **338**: 293–5.

Kendell RE, Chalmers JC, Platz C (1987) Epidemiology of puerperal psychoses. *British Journal of Psychiatry*, **150**: 662–73.

Kim JJ, Gean AD (2011) Imaging for the diagnosis and management of traumatic brain injury. *Neurotherapeutics*, **8**: 39–53.

Kingham M, Gordon H (2004) Aspects of morbid jealousy. *Advances in Psychiatric Treatment*, **10**: 207–15.

Kipps CM, Hodges JR (2008) Clinical cognitive assessment. In *Oxford Textbook of Old Age Psychiatry* (eds R Jacoby, C Oppenheimer, T Denning, *et al*). Oxford University Press.

Kleber HD (2007) Pharmacologic treatments for opioid dependence: detoxification and maintenance options. *Dialogues in Clinical Neuroscience*, **9**: 455–70.

Koran LM (2007) Obsessive–compulsive disorder. An update for the clinician. *Focus*, **5**: 299–313.

Lai M-C, Lombardo MV, Baron-Cohen S (2014) Autism. *Lancet*, **383**: 896–910.

Lally J, Higaya E-E, Nisar Z, *et al* (2013) Prevalence study of head shop drug usage in mental health services. *The Psychiatrist*, **37**: 44–8.

Lasserre AM, Glaus J, Vandeleur CL, *et al* (2014) Depression with atypical features and increase in obesity, body mass index, waist circumference, and fat mass: a prospective, population-based study. *JAMA Psychiatry*, **71**: 880–8.

Leichsenring F, Leibling E, Kruse J, et al (2011) Borderline personality disorder. *Lancet*, **377**: 74–84.

Leucht S, Heres S (2006) Epidemiology, clinical consequences, and psychosocial treatment of nonadherence in schizophrenia. *Journal of Clinical Psychiatry*, **5**: 3–8.

Leucht S, Burkard T, Henderson J, et al (2007) Physical illness and schizophrenia: a review of the literature. *Acta Psychiatrica Scandinavica*, **116**: 317–33.

Leucht S, Corves C, Arbter D, et al (2009) Second generation versus first generation antipsychotic drugs for schizophrenia: a meta-analysis. *Lancet*, **373**: 31–41.

Levy KN (2005) The implications of attachment theory and research for understanding borderline personality disorder. *Development and Psychopathology*, **17**: 959.

Lieberman JA, Koreen AR, Chakos M, et al (1996) Factors influencing treatment response and outcome of first-episode schizophrenia: implications for understanding the pathophysiology of schizophrenia. *Journal of Clinical Psychiatry*, **57** (Suppl 9): 5–9.

Lieberman JA, Stroup TS, McEvoy JP, et al (2005) Effectiveness of antipsychotic drugs in patients with chronic schizophrenia. *New England Journal of Medicine*, **353**: 1209–23.

Lincoln TM, Wilhelm K, Nestoriuc Y (2007) Effectiveness of psychoeducation for relapse, symptoms, knowledge, adherence and functioning in psychotic disorders: a meta-analysis. *Schizophrenia Research*, **96**: 232–45.

Linscott RJ, van Os J (2013) An updated and conservative systematic review and meta-analysis of epidemiological evidence on psychotic experiences in children and adults: on the pathway from proneness to persistence to dimensional expression across mental disorders. *Psychological Medicine*, **43**: 1133–49.

Lynch D, Laws KR, McKenna PJ (2010) Cognitive behavioural therapy for major psychiatric disorder: does it really work? A meta-analytical review of well-controlled trials. *Psychological Medicine*, **40**: 9–24.

Malhi GS, Hitching R, Berk M, et al (2013) Pharmacological management of unipolar depression. *Acta Psychiatrica Scandinavica Supplementaum*, **443**: 6–23.

Mancebo MC, Eisen JL, Grant JE, et al (2005) Obsessive compulsive personality disorder and obsessive compulsive disorder: clinical characteristics, diagnostic difficulties, and treatment. *Annals of Clinical Psychiatry*, **17**: 197–204.

Mannarino AP, Cohen JA, Deblinger E (2014) Trauma-focused cognitive–behavioral therapy. In *Evidence-Based Approaches for the Treatment of Maltreated Children* (eds S Timmer, A Urquiza). Springer.

Martin GN, Carlson NR, Busskist W (2013) *Psychology* (5th edn). Pearson.

Maust DT, Kim HM, Seyfried LS, et al (2015) Antipsychotics, other psychotropics, and the risk of death in patients with dementia: number needed to harm. *JAMA Psychiatry*, **72**: 438–45.

McEvoy JP, Lieberman JA, Stroup TS, et al (2006) Effectiveness of clozapine versus olanzapine, quetiapine, and risperidone in patients with chronic schizophrenia who did not respond to prior atypical antipsychotic treatment. *American Journal of Psychiatry*, **163**: 600–10.

McGrath J, Saha S, Chant D, et al (2008) Schizophrenia: a concise overview of incidence, prevalence, and mortality. *Epidemiologic Reviews*, **30**: 67–76.

McKee AC, Cantu RC, Nowinski CJ, et al (2009) Chronic traumatic encephalopathy in athletes: progressive tauopathy following repetitive head injury. *Journal of Neuropathology and Experimental Neurology*, **68**: 709–35.

McKeith I, Mintzer J, Aarsland D, et al (2004) Dementia with Lewy bodies. *Lancet Neurology*, **3**: 19–28.

McKeith IG, Dickson DW, Lowe J, et al (2005) Diagnosis and management of dementia with Lewy bodies: third report of the DLB Consortium. *Neurology*, **65**: 1863–72.

McKnight RF, Adida M, Budge K, et al (2012) Lithium toxicity profile: a systematic review and meta-analysis. *Lancet*, **379**: 721–8.

Meagher D, Leonard M (2008) The active management of delirium: improving detection and treatment. *Advances in Psychiatric Treatment*, **14**: 292–301.

Mellers JDC (2009) Epilepsy. In *Lishman's Organic Psychiatry: A Textbook of Neuropsychiatry* (4th edn) (eds A David, S Fleminger, M Kopelman, *et al*). Wiley–Blackwell.

Mintz AR, Dobson KS, Romney DM (2003) Insight in schizophrenia: a meta-analysis. *Schizophrenia Research*, **61**: 75–88.

Mitchell AJ, Vancampfort D, Sweers K, *et al* (2013) Prevalence of metabolic syndrome and metabolic abnormalities in schizophrenia and related disorders – a systematic review and meta-analysis. *Schizophrenia Bulletin*, **39**: 306–18.

Mittal, VA, Kalus O, Bernstein DP, *et al* (2007) Schizoid personality disorder. In *Personality Disorders: Toward the DSM-V* (eds LJ Siever, W O'Donohue, KA Fowler, *et al*). Sage.

Mizuno Y, Suzuki T, Nakagawa A, *et al* (2014) Pharmacological strategies to counteract antipsychotic-induced weight gain and metabolic adverse effects in schizophrenia: a systematic review and meta-analysis. *Schizophrenia Bulletin*, doi: 10.1093/schbul/sbu030.

Moore TH, Zammit S, Lingford-Hughes A, *et al* (2007) Cannabis use and risk of psychotic or affective mental health outcomes: a systematic review. *Lancet*, **370**: 319–28.

Moran M (2013) New gender dysphoria criteria replace GID. *Psychiatric News*, doi: 10.1176/appi.pn.2013.4a19.

Morgan C, Charalambides M, Hutchinson G, *et al* (2010) Migration, ethnicity, and psychosis: toward a sociodevelopmental model. *Schizophrenia Bulletin*, **36**: 655–64.

Mueser KT, Bellack AS, Brady EU (1990) Hallucinations in schizophrenia. *Acta Psychiatrica Scandinavica*, **82**: 26–9.

Musters C, McDonald E, Jones L (2008) Management of postnatal depression. *BMJ*, **337**: 399–403.

Nardell M, Tampi RR (2014) Pharmacological treatments for frontotemporal dementias: a systematic review of randomized controlled trials. *American Journal of Alzheimer's Disease and Other Dementias*, **29**: 123–32.

NHS Choices (2013) Post-traumatic stress disorder – treatment (PTSD). *NHS Choices* (http://www.nhs.uk/Conditions/Post-traumatic-stress-disorder/Pages/Treatment.aspx).

NICE (2004) *Eating Disorders: Core Interventions in the Treatment and Management of Anorexia Nervosa, Bulimia Nervosa and Related Eating Disorders* (CG9). NICE.

NICE (2007) *Drug Misuse: Psychosocial Interventions* (CG51). NICE.

NICE (2008) *Attention Deficit Hyperactivity Disorder: Diagnosis and Management of ADHD in Children, Young People and Adults* (CG72). NICE.

NICE (2009*a*) *Depression in Adults: The Treatment and Management of Depression in Adults* (CG90). NICE.

NICE (2009*b*) *Antenatal and Postnatal Mental Health: Clinical Management and Service Guidance* (CG192). NICE.

NICE (2010) *Alcohol-Use Disorders: Diagnosis and Clinical Management of Alcohol-Related Physical Complications* (CG100). NICE.

NICE (2011*a*) *Alcohol-Use Disorders: Diagnosis, Assessment and Management of Harmful Drinking and Alcohol Dependence* (CG115). NICE.

NICE (2011*b*) *Donepezil, galantamine, rivastigmine and memantine for the treatment of Alzheimer's disease* (TA217). NICE.

NICE (2014) *Pscyhosis and Schizophrenia in Adults: Treatment and Management* (CG178). NICE.

Nicholson TRJ, Cutter W, Hotopf M (2008) Assessing mental capacity: The Mental Capacity Act. *BMJ*, **336**: 322.

Nielsen J, Graff C, Kanters JK, *et al* (2011) Assessing QT interval prolongation and its associated risks with antipsychotics. *CNS Drugs*, **25**: 473–90.

Nordgaard J, Arnfred SM, Handest P, *et al* (2008) The diagnostic status of first-rank symptoms. *Schizophrenia Bulletin*, **34**: 137–54.

O'Connell H, Kennelly SP, Cullen W, *et al* (2014) Managing delirium in everyday practice: towards cognitive-friendly hospitals. *Advances in Psychiatric Treatment*, **20**: 380–9.

O'Donnell ML, Alkemade N, Nickerson A, *et al* (2014) Impact of the diagnostic changes to post-traumatic stress disorder for DSM-5 and the proposed changes to ICD-11. *British Journal of Psychiatry*, **205**: 230–5.

Oyebode F (2008) *Sims' Symptoms in the Mind: An Introduction to Descriptive Psychopathology*. Elsevier.

Oyebode F (2013) Karl Jaspers: 100 years of General Psychopathology – reflection. *British Journal of Psychiatry*, **203**: 405.

Ozonoff S, Young GS, Carter A, *et al* (2011) Recurrence risk for autism spectrum disorders: a Baby Siblings Research Consortium Study. *Pediatrics*, **128**: e1–8.

Parmelee PA, Katz IR (1990) Geriatric Depression Scale; to the Editor. *Journal of the American Geriatrics Society*, **38**: 1379.

Pasquier F, Deramecourt V, Lebert F (2008) Frontotemporal dementia. In *Oxford Textbook of Old Age Psychiatry* (eds R Jacoby, C Oppenheimer, T Denning, *et al*). Oxford University Press.

Pelkonen M, Marttunen M (2003) Child and adolescent suicide: epidemiology, risk factors, and approaches to prevention. *Paediatric Drugs*, **5**: 243–65.

Perry EC (2014) Inpatient management of acute alcohol withdrawal syndrome. *CNS Drugs*, **28**: 401–10.

Pompili M, Serafini G, Innamorati M, *et al* (2011) Suicide risk in first episode psychosis: a selective review of the current literature. *Schizophrenia Research*, **129**: 1–11.

Raylu N, Oei TP (2002) Pathological gambling: a comprehensive review. *Clinical Psychology Review*, **22**: 1009–61.

Robertson E, Grace S, Wallington T, *et al* (2004) Antenatal risk factors for postpartum depression: a synthesis of recent literature. *General Hospital Psychiatry*, **26**: 289–95.

Rogers R (ed) (2008) *Clinical Assessment of Malingering and Deception*. Guilford Press.

Rosen C, Grossman LS, Harrow M, *et al* (2011) Diagnostic and prognostic significance of Schneiderian first-rank symptoms: a 20-year longitudinal study of schizophrenia and bipolar disorder. *Comprehensive Psychiatry*, **52**: 126–31.

Rothbaum BO, Meadows EA, Resick P, *et al* (2000) Cognitive–behavioral therapy. In *Effective Treatments for PTSD: Practice Guidelines from the International Society for Traumatic Stress Studies* (eds EB Foa, TM Keane, MJ Friedman). Guilford Press.

Royal College of Psychiatrists (2013) *Anxiety, Panic and Phobias*. Royal College of Psychiatrists (www.rcpsych.ac.uk/healthadvice/problemsdisorders/anxiety,panic,phobias.aspx).

Saunders KEA, Goodwin GM (2010) The course of bipolar disorder. *Advances in Psychiatric Treatment*, **16**: 318–28.

Schneider LS, Insel PS, Weiner MW, *et al* (2011) Treatment with cholinesterase inhibitors and memantine of patients in the Alzheimer's Disease Neuroimaging Initiative. *Archives of Neurology*, **68**: 58–66.

Schorr SG, Slooff CJ, Postema R, *et al* (2008) A 12-month follow-up study of treating overweight schizophrenic patients with aripiprazole. *Acta Psychiatrica Scandinavica*, **118**: 246–50.

Schou M (1997) Forty years of lithium treatment. *Archives of General Psychiatry*, **54**: 9–13.

Schrank B, Slade M (2007) Recovery in psychiatry. *Psychiatric Bulletin*, **31**: 321–5.

Semple D, Smyth, R (2013*a*) Eating and impulse-control disorders. In *Oxford Handbook of Psychiatry* (eds D Semple, R Smyth). Oxford University Press.

Semple D, Smyth R (2013*b*) Transcultural psychiatry. In *Oxford Handbook of Psychiatry* (eds D Semple, R Smyth). Oxford University Press.

Shapiro F, Laliotis D (2010) EMDR and the adaptive information processing model: Integrative treatment and case conceptualization. *Clinical Social Work Journal*, **39**: 191–200.

Shapiro JR, Berkman ND, Browley KA, *et al* (2007) Bulimia nervosa treatment: a systematic review of randomized controlled trials. *International Journal of Eating Disorders*, **40**: 321–36.

Sharpley MS, Hutchinson G, Murray RM, *et al* (2001) Understanding the excess of psychosis among the African-Caribbean population in England. Review of current hypotheses. *British Journal of Psychiatry*, **40** (Suppl): s60–8.

Shimizu M, Kubota Y, Toichi M, *et al* (2007) Folie à deux and shared psychotic disorder. *Current Psychiatry Reports*, **9**: 200–5.

Sikich L, Frazier JA, McClellan J, *et al* (2008) Double-blind comparison of first- and second-generation antipsychotics in early-onset schizophrenia and schizoaffective disorder: findings from the treatment of early-onset schizophrenia spectrum disorders (TEOSS) study. *American Journal of Psychiatry*, **165**: 1420–31.

Sims A (2012) *Religious Delusions*. Royal College of Psychiatrists (https://www.rcpsych.ac.uk/pdf/Religious%20delusions%20Andrew%20Sims.pdf).

Smiley E (2005) Epidemiology of mental health problems in adults with learning disability: an update. *Advances in Psychiatric Treatment*, **11**: 214–22.

Smink FR, van Hoeken D, Hoek HW (2012) Epidemiology of eating disorders: incidence, prevalence and mortality rates. *Current Psychiatry Reports*, **14**: 406–14.

Smith D, Jones I, Simpson S (2010) Psychoeducation for bipolar disorder. *Advances in Psychiatric Treatment*, **16**: 147–54.

Snowdon J (2011) Pseudodementia, a term for its time: the impact of Leslie Kiloh's 1961 paper. *Australasian Psychiatry*, **19**: 391–7.

Spencer E, Birchwood M, McGovern D (2001) Management of first-episode psychosis. *Advances in Psychiatric Treatment*, **7**: 133–40.

Stanton LR, Coetzee RH (2004) Down's syndrome and dementia. *Advances in Psychiatric Treatment*, **10**: 50–8.

Starcevic V (2012) Benzodiazepines for anxiety disorders: maximising the benefits and minimising the risks. *Advances in Psychiatric Treatment*, **18**: 250–8.

Stevens A (2001) *Jung: A Very Short Introduction*. Oxford University Press.

Stewart R (2008) Vascular and mixed dementia. In *Oxford Textbook of Old Age Psychiatry* (eds R Jacoby, C Oppenheimer, T Denning, *et al*). Oxford University Press.

Stoffers JM, Vollm BA, Rucker G *et al* (2012) Psychological therapies for people with borderline personality disorder. *Cochrane Database Systematic Reviews*, **8**: CD005652.

Stompe T, Ortwein-Swoboda G, Schanda H (2004) Schizophrenia, delusional symptoms, and violence: The threat/control-override concept reexamined. *Schizophrenia Bulletin*, **30**: 31.

Stone J, Carson A, Sharpe M (2005) Functional symptoms and signs in neurology: assessment and diagnosis. *Journal of Neurology, Neurosurgery and Psychiatry*, **76**: i2–12.

Storr A (2001) *Freud: A Very Short Introduction*. Oxford University Press.

Swinkels WA, Kuyk J, van Dyck R, *et al* (2005) Psychiatric comorbidity in epilepsy. *Epilepsy and Behavior*, **7**: 37–50.

Talley NJ, O'Connor S (2010) *Clinical Examination: A Systematic Guide to Physical Diagnosis*. Elsevier.

Taylor D, Paton C, Kapur S (2012) *The Maudsley Prescribing Guidelines in Psychiatry*. Wiley.

Thom M, Bertram EH (2011) Temporal lobe epilepsy. *Handbook of Clinical Neurology*, **107**: 225–40.

Thomas A (2008) Alzheimer's disease. In *Oxford Textbook of Old Age Psychiatry* (eds R Jacoby, C Oppenheimer, T Denning, *et al*). Oxford University Press.

Thornicroft G, Tansella M (2005) Growing recognition of the importance of service user involvement in mental health service planning and evaluation. *Epidemiologia e Psichiatria Sociale*, **14**: 1–3.

Tomson T, Xue H, Battino D (2015) Major congenital malformations in children of women with epilepsy. *Seizure*, **28**: 46–50.

Triebwasser J, Chemerinski E, Roussos P, *et al* (2012) Schizoid personality disorder. *Journal of Personality Disorders*, **26**: 919–26.

Triebwasser J, Chemerinski E, Roussos P, *et al* (2013) Paranoid personality disorder. *Journal of Personality Disorders*, **27**: 795–805.

Tyrer P, Crawford M, Mulder R, *et al* (2011) The rationale for the reclassification of personality disorder in the 11th revision of the International Classification of Diseases (ICD-11). *Personality and Mental Health*, **5**: 246–59.

Vahia IV, Palmer BW, Depp C, *et al* (2010) Is late-onset schizophrenia a subtype of schizophrenia? *Acta Psychiatrica Scandinavica*, **122**: 414–26.

Vancampfort D, Stubbs B, Mitchell AJ, *et al* (2015) Risk of metabolic syndrome and its components in people with schizophrenia and related psychotic disorders, bipolar disorder and major depressive disorder: a systematic review and meta-analysis. *World Psychiatry*, **14**: 339–47.

Van der Zwaard R, Polak MA (2001) Pseudohallucinations: A pseudoconcept? A review of the validity of the concept, related to associate symptomatology. *Comprehensive Psychiatry*, **42**: 42–50.

Van Gastel WA, MacCabe JH, Schubart CD, *et al* (2013) Cigarette smoking and cannabis use are equally strongly associated with psychotic-like experiences: a cross-sectional study in 1929 young adults. *Psychological Medeicine*, **43**: 2393–401.

Varma S, Bishara D, Besag FMC, *et al* (2011) Clozapine-related EEG changes and seizures: dose and plasma-level relationships. *Therapeutic Advances in Psychopharmacology*, **1**: 47–66.

Velamoor VR (1998) Neuroleptic malignant syndrome. Recognition, prevention and management. *Drug Safety*, **19**: 73–82.

Viswanathan A, Rocca WA, Tzourio C (2009) Vascular risk factors and dementia: how to move forward? *Neurology*, **72**: 368–74.

Vriends N, Bolt OC, Kunz SM (2014) Social anxiety disorder, a lifelong disorder? A review of the spontaneous remission and its predictors. *Acta Psychiatrica Scandinavica*, **130**: 109–22.

Wakefield JC, Schmitz MF (2013) Normal vs. disordered bereavement-related depression: are the differences real or tautological? *Acta Psychiatrica Scandinavica*, **127**: 159–68.

Wenk GL (2003) Neuropathologic changes in Alzheimer's disease. *Journal of Clinical Psychiatry*, **64** (Suppl 9): 7–10.

Whyte IM, Francis B, Dawson AH (2007) Safety and efficacy of intravenous N-acetylcysteine for acetaminophen overdose: analysis of the Hunter Area Toxicology Service (HATS) database. *Current Medical Research and Opinion*, **23**: 2359–68.

Wilkinson P, Izmeth Z (2012) Continuation and maintenance treatments for depression in older people. *Cochrane Database of Systematic Reviews*, **11**: CD00672.

World Health Organization (1992) *The ICD-10 Classification of Mental and Behavioural Disorders. Clinical Descriptions and Diagnostic Guidelines*. WHO.

Index

Compiled by Linda English

tremor 66, 77, 85, 93, 136, 142, 151, 152, 154
tricyclic antidepressants 49, 88, 140, 146, 147, 149, 160, 161
12-step programs 64–65, 73

urban living 21, 31
urea 147, 161

Valliant, George 168
varencline 64, 73
vascular dementia 77, 84, 85
venlafaxine 49, 146, 160

violence 108, 177, 184, 189
  risk of 12, 13, 40, 175, 180–181, 184, 189, 194
visual hallucinations 14, 15, 68, 75, 82, 93, 94, 128, 136, 143, 154
visuospatial skills test 81, 92

waist circumference 126, 134
weight gain
  antipsychotics 124, 130, 131, 132, 134, 139, 140, 148
  atypical depression 128, 137
Wernicke's encephalopathy 62, 67, 69–70
working memory 7, 15
World War II: naming dates 81, 92